The Skin

Cancer

Answer

Dr. I. William Lane
Linda Comac

AVERY PUBLISHING GROUP

Garden City Park • New York

The therapeutic procedures in this book are based on the training, personal experiences, and research of the authors. Because each person and situation is unique, the authors and publisher urge the reader to check with a qualified health professional before using any procedure where there is any question to appropriateness.

The publisher does not advocate the use of any particular health treatment, but believes the information presented in this book should be available to the public. Because there is always some risk involved, the author and publisher are not responsible for any adverse effects or consequences resulting from the use of any of the suggestions, preparations, or procedures described in this book. Please do not use the book if you are unwilling to assume the risk. Feel free to consult with a physician or other qualified health professional. It is a sign of wisdom, not cowardice, to seek a second or third opinion.

Cover Designer: Eric Macaluso
In-House Editor: Marie Caratozzolo
Typesetter: Helen Contoudis
Printer: Paragon Press, Honesdale, PA

Avery Publishing Group
120 Old Broadway
Garden City Park, NY 11040
1–800–548–5757

Library of Congress Cataloging-in-Publication Data

Lane, I. William
     The skin cancer answer : the natural treatment for basal and
squamous cell carcinomas and keratoses / I. William Lane & Linda
Comac.
            p.   cm.
     Includes bibliographical references and index.
     ISBN 0–89529–865–1
     1. Skin Cancer—Alternative treatment. 2. Glycoalkaloids—Therapeutic use.
3. Solanum—Therapeutic use. I. Comac, Linda.
  II. Title.
  RC280.S5L36   1999
  616.99′47706—dc21   99–31180
                                                 CIP

Printed in the United States of America

10 9 8 7 6 5 4 3 2 1

Contents

Acknowledgments

A special thanks goes to David Williams for bringing this work to my attention and to the Australian scientists who made it all possible. Recognition must also go to Joni Mitchell and Lorna Goshman of the University of Wisconsin School of Pharmacy for their invaluable assistance in locating information for this book. On a final note, I would like to thank all the dedicated research scientists who believe in Nature's ability to heal.

Preface

Questions and problems abound. Whether discussing the economy, race relations, or global warming, we are confronted with situations whose remedies seem to require the wisdom of Solomon. Fortunately, every age, every field has its Solomons—men and women like Dr. Martin Luther King, Jr., Louis Pasteur, Albert Einstein, Marie Curie, and Horace Mann. Because thoughtful, innovative people walk among us, solutions to some of the world's most pressing problems may be at hand.

We have, for instance, long lived in fear that our depleted ozone layer would result in skin cancer for many of us and for our loved ones. Indeed, the rates for adolescents and the elderly are considered epidemic. Thankfully, there is now evidence that international efforts to ban the use of various chemicals is beginning to have a positive effect. Some researchers predict that the ozone layer will be repaired at the start of the twenty-first century. But for those who already have skin cancer, this is a small consolation.

These people can only hope that the cut, burn, and poison remedies of allopathic medicine can prevent their cancers from spreading. If their cancers are found early, they can look forward to trading their disease for permanent and often disfiguring scars and to incurring the risk of infection, bleeding, and anesthesia-induced mortality. Until now.

Now researchers in Australia—birthplace of heart-transplant surgery and center of the highest incidence of skin cancer on the planet—have made discoveries that promise to trade surgery, chemotherapy, and radiation treatment for a simple topical application of chemicals derived from plants. That's right, an effective all-natural skin cancer treatment has been derived from common, everyday vegetables in the genus *Solanum*.

While traveling in Australia investigating a new method for processing shark cartilage, David G. Williams, D.C., learned about a simple cream that was reported to eliminate skin cancers. As soon as Dave told me of his discovery, I realized that the findings had to come up from "down under." And now they have arrived.

In *The Skin Cancer Answer*, I'll tell you how grave your risk of contracting skin cancer really is and why. In Part One, we'll look at our planet, ourselves, and our relationship with the sun. You'll see how destruction of the ozone layer has resulted in an increased incidence of skin cancer.

Once you've finished the background material in Part One, *The Skin Cancer Answer* will give you an in-depth look at "The Problem—Skin Cancer" in Part Two. Here you'll learn about the causes and various types of skin cancer, the difficulties involved in trying to prevent the condition, and the problem-laden treatments currently being offered. We'll examine the success rate of various treatments and look at the side effects associated with each.

In Part Three, we'll look into "The Answer—Glycoalkaloids," a technical-sounding name for extracts from absolutely common plants with absolutely extraordinary abilities. You'll find out exactly what these extracts are, how they are made, and how they work. We'll look at current research from around the world that daily provides new evidence on the effectiveness of the glycoalkaloid preparations. You'll find out that extracts from plants in the genus *Solanum* have decided advantages over the established treatments of surgery, chemotherapy, and radiation. And just in case the concept of an effective natural skin cancer treatment leaves you a bit skeptical, I'll take you on a quick tour of time-honored plant-derived medicinals such as digitalis, aspirin, and sudephedrine.

As you turn the pages of *The Skin Cancer Answer*, you will discover information that has been too long hidden from the American public. Come with me and learn how you can find healing in the fruits of the field—healing that is pain- and risk-free.

Introduction

Since Adam and Eve ate the apple from the tree of knowledge, people have been making mistakes. Sometimes people make mistakes because, like Adam and Eve, they don't follow important instructions or advice. Sometimes they make mistakes because they act too quickly, reaching out for a tempting treat without weighing the consequences.

The story of skin cancer is a story of mistakes. It is the story of a technology that people grabbed at without adequate planning. The temptations of cool rooms in the summer, strong disposable plates, and products dispensed by the touch of a button led us into the widespread use of chlorofluorocarbons (CFCs). No one suspected CFCs would destroy the ozone layer, leaving people at increased risk for skin cancer. And the lure of the sun—deliciously warm and bright—is proving too strong a temptation to resist. Too many people succumb to the sun's allure, ignoring the warnings about excessive exposure.

But humankind is also tempted to rise above its errors. The same inquisitiveness and impatience that drives mankind to make mistakes inspires solutions. Cast out of the Garden of Eden, Adam and Eve donned fig leaves and went to work planting crops. Faced with a hole in the ozone layer and increasing skin cancer rates, twentieth-century people are looking for—and finding—solutions.

CONFRONTING THE PROBLEM

Melanoma—the most lethal of the skin cancers—is occurring more and more frequently. In 1935, a person's lifetime risk of developing melanoma was 1 in 1,500. By 1980, that risk had increased to 1 in 250. By the year 2000, the risk will be 1 in 75! It is now estimated that 50 percent of people who reach the age of sixty-five will develop some form of skin cancer. Not only is the incidence of the disease increasing, but death rates from malignant melanomas have increased in white males and females.

And melanoma is just one type of skin cancer. When melanoma and nonmelanoma skin cancers are combined, skin cancer is seen as the most common tumorous condition in the United States. The number of nonmelanoma skin cancers—referred to as squamous and basal cell carcinomas—is actually equal to the number of cancers that occur at all other sites combined.

Why is modern man so plagued by skin cancers? The answer is quite simple—too much exposure to sunlight! But it may be even easier to solve this problem than it was for Adam and Eve to solve theirs. You don't need to don a fig leaf or plant a crop. You don't even have to leave your garden. Just read on.

Part One

Sunlight—A Mixed Blessing

Melanoma of the skin is virtually epidemic
among both young adults and the elderly.

Dr. Barney Kernet and Patricia Lawler
Your Skin: Prevention, Early Detection, and
Treatment of Melanoma and Other Skin Cancers

"The sun will come up tomorrow . . ." so sings
Annie in the musical production based on the
famous comic strip character. Her song has
come to be the anthem of optimism, for surely
if the sun shines, all is right with the world. There is warmth and
brightness, plants grow, and the food chain thrives. But . . .

There is a flip side to the glittering image of sunlight. There
is solar radiation, sunburn, and sunspots. There is the fear that
the ozone layer will continue to diminish, exposing us to too
much sun. Too much sun—most of us have learned through
painful experience—is not a good thing. And as time and technology have moved forward, the specter of a world literally
plagued by too much sunshine has moved from the realm of science fiction into the realm of scientific journals.

Researchers, physicians, and most of the general public are now convinced that skin cancers are the direct result of exposure to sunlight. "The incidence of squamous and basal cell carcinomas of the skin in fair white-skinned persons is directly related to the amount of yearly sunlight in the area," claims *The Merck Manual*. And a report by the United States Office of Technology Assessment claims, "There is no doubt that natural radiation, consisting of ionizing radiation from cosmic rays and radioactive materials, can cause cancer. . . . Ultraviolet radiation from the Sun is believed responsible for most of the 400,000 non-melanoma skin cancers." The same report lists "Radiation, ultraviolet" as an "Occupational Cancer Hazard" for farmers,

Sun Facts

- *The sun is 865,000 miles in diameter; 1.3 million Earths would fit inside it.*
- *The sun has been shining for 5 billion years.*
- *The temperature on the sun's surface is 10,832°F.*
- *The temperature at the sun's core is 27,000,000°F.*
- *More than 30 percent of the sun's rays are reflected back into space.*
- *More than two-thirds of the sun's radiation is absorbed by the atmosphere, clouds, and the Earth's surface.*
- *The sun is 93 million miles from the Earth.*
- *The planets in our solar system are pulled around the sun by gravitation and circle it in extended circular paths called "ellipses." The speed of the planets varies according to their distance from the sun.*

sailors, and arc welders. What is it about life-affirming sun-beams that can also prove deadly?

At the center of the sun, the temperature is hot enough—27,000,000°F—for hydrogen atoms to fuse into helium atoms in the process known as hydrogen fusion. It is almost as if the sun is a huge hydrogen bomb exploding in space. During the fusion process, energy is released in the form of gamma rays that move outward in all directions. As the gamma rays move out from the core to the sun's surface, they become visible rays of light and other forms of solar radiation such as ultraviolet light, which is invisible. Visible light is just a small percentage of the whole range of radiation, which is known as the electromagnetic spec-trum and includes gamma rays, x-rays, infrared radiation, radio waves, and microwaves.

All these different forms of radiation are characterized by the length of their waves. Ultraviolet (UV) rays measure from about 4 to 380 nanometers (nm). A nanometer is one billionth of a meter. UV-B rays measure from about 280 to 320 nm, while UV-A rays are approximately 320 to 380 nm. UV-C rays are 10 to 280 nm. Only UV-A and UV-B rays reach the surface of the Earth. The rays that produce sunburns are those below 320 nm—UV-B rays.

In moderation, UV-B rays induce tanning, a process that helps to protect the skin from too much exposure to sunlight by thickening the epidermis and causing an increase in pigmenta-tion. The action of these rays on the ergosterol present in human skin produces vitamin D, but the same rays that have such a positive effect can also have deleterious effects.

Excessive exposure to UV rays causes sunburn. The leathery, wrinkled skin of many sun worshippers attests to the aging effect of constant exposure to sunlight. Experts agree that pre-cancerous skin lesions are a frequent disturbing consequence of overexposure to the sun.

Nuclear fusion reactions within the sun produce energy that reaches the Earth as visible radiation and invisible radiation.

Let There Be Light

Creation stories the world over are full of references to light. In Genesis in the Old Testament, the Lord says, "Let there be Light." In the creation myth from the Kono people of Guinea, all is darkness until the tou-tou bird and the rooster are given a son "to call forth the light of day." The Maidu Indians in California have an origin myth in which the god Earth Starter tells his sister to come up in the east. In Australia, the Northern Aranda aborigines tell the tale of Karora, the Creator who lay asleep in the forever darkness until the sun rose at Ilbalintja. And in a creation myth from the Quiche Maya of Guatemala, there was darkness within which were the Maker and the Feathered Serpent who were glittered with light.

Light seems to be a universal symbol of beginnings. We know, too, that it is a symbol of hope and of knowledge. Yet mankind's knowledge of light itself is a relatively new science and our understanding of light is still far from complete.

The Islamic scientist Ibn al-Haytham (965–c.1040) may have been the first to understand the nature of light. He rejected the Greek concept that the eye sends out rays of light to objects at which it looks. He believed instead that rays of light come from the object to the eye. He also studied lenses and decided that bending or refraction of light is caused by rays moving at different speeds through different materials.

Many years later, Sir Isaac Newton, the famous seventeenth-century British scientist who postulated the theory of gravity, conducted experiments with light. Directing a beam of sunlight through a glass prism, he noted that the light was split into shades ranging from violet to red. This experiment demonstrated that sunlight is a mixture of red, orange, yellow, green, blue, indigo, and violet — that famous mnemonic "ROY G. BIV."

In 1895, the German scientist Wilhelm Roentgen conducted research on cathode rays, produced when electricity is passed through a glass tube that holds a near-vacuum. When Roentgen completely surrounded the tube with black paper, a cardboard on the other side of the room glowed. The cardboard, which had been coated with a fluorescent chemical that glows in the light, glowed even when moved to the next room. Roentgen deduced that the tube was emitting a form of radiation that could pass through various materials. He named this form of radiation "x-rays" because their origin was unknown.

Roentgen subsequently found that x-rays enabled him to take photographs that revealed the bones inside the human body. The rays could not pass through the bones but did pass through the flesh, allowing the photographic image to be formed.

French physicist Antoine Becquerel, who was studying a fluorescent compound that included uranium, was fascinated by Roentgen's discovery. He wrapped the uranium in metal foil and put it on a photographic plate to find if a fluorescent chemical would emit x-rays. Upon developing the plate, he discovered it had been blackened so it was obviously emitting some kind of ray. Later experiments showed that the blackening occurred with uranium but not other fluorescent chemicals. Becquerel deduced that the substance was sending out a particularly strong type of radiation. Eventually, it was determined that there are three types of radiation: alpha and beta, which consist of electrically charged particles, and gamma, a form of electromagnetic radiation.

Marya Sklodowska, a Polish chemist who studied in Paris where she met and married the chemist Pierre Curie, also conducted research into radiation. The Curies experimented with pitchblende, a mineral that contains uranium but is four times as radioactive as that substance. They purified an unknown element and named it "radium." This element, which in small doses is medically useful, can be dangerous. Because of constant exposure to radium over many years, Marie Curie developed leukemia from which she died in 1934.

Today, we know that radiation causes cancer, including skin cancers that result from excessive UV exposure. Research has also revealed that excessive exposure to the sun promotes wrinkles and cataracts. A great deal of modern research focuses on light as a mixed blessing—warming and brightening even as it destroys.

Most of this is converted to heat when it strikes the ground. The sun's rays, therefore, warm anything they touch. Without these rays, the Earth would be a barren wasteland, too cold to support life. Even if there were enough warmth without sunlight, there still would be no food to eat. Through the process called *photosynthesis*, green plants use the energy from the sun's rays to convert water and carbon dioxide into the carbohydrates they need for food. Without sunlight, there would be no green plants, and without green plants, there would be no food for animals to eat. Of course, if there were too much sunlight—if, for instance, the Earth got too close to the sun—everything would be burned to a crisp. Right now the sun is 93 million miles from Earth—just the right distance.

SHIELDED FROM THE SUN

Although the Earth's distance from the sun has remained unchanged, the amount of rays reaching Earth has, unfortunately, increased. Under optimal conditions, the atmosphere—a 430-mile-thick layer of gas surrounding Earth—acts as a protective shield. Here, meteors burn up before they can strike the Earth's surface and harmful rays of the sun are absorbed.

The atmosphere actually consists of four layers: the troposphere, stratosphere, mesosphere, and thermosphere, as shown in Figure 1.1 on page 10. In the upper layers of the atmosphere is the ozone layer, a belt of gasses ten to thirty miles above the Earth's surface. When intact, the ozone layer absorbs 99 percent of the ultraviolet-B (UV-B) radiation, which amounts to less than 5 percent of the sun's radiation. The ozone layer is thickest twelve to nineteen miles above the Earth's surface in the stratosphere. Because the ozone layer was significantly reduced between 1979 and 1992—as much as 40 percent—in heavily populated areas of the Northern hemisphere, there has been a 6 percent increase in the number of UV-B rays reaching the Earth.

The ozone layer is our first line of defense against overexposure to the sun. In addition to being absorbed by the ozone layer, UV-B rays below 320 nm—those that can cause sunburn—are also absorbed by air impurities such as water, smoke, and dust, as well as ordinary window glass.

ABOUT THE OZONE LAYER

Today, we are all aware that there is a hole in the ozone layer. Few of us, however, seem to know just what ozone is.

Ozone is actually a form of oxygen. As you know, oxygen is a gas, and all gases are comprised of atoms grouped into molecules. One oxygen molecule has two atoms of oxygen (O_2).

When the sun's rays hit the stratosphere, these atoms become separated. Once the oxygen molecule has been separated, a free oxygen atom can join an intact oxygen molecule to form ozone, which consists of three atoms of oxygen (O_3). The ozone is formed when oxygen absorbs the energy from the ultraviolet radiation. For this reason, ozone levels vary according to the number and strength of the sun's rays that reach Earth. Ozone is an unstable gas; its atoms separate easily and can then join with other atoms and molecules to form either oxygen or ozone.

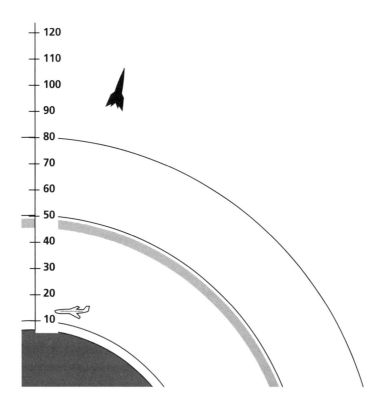

Figure 1.1. The Layers of the Earth's Atmosphere

Destruction of the Ozone Layer

The presence of chemicals such as chlorine and bromine in the upper atmosphere interferes with the natural balance of ozone. Chlorine atoms are released into the atmosphere by chlorofluorocarbons (CFCs) that rise into the stratosphere. These chlorine atoms then break down the ozone layer by pulling off one atom of oxygen and forming chlorine monoxide (C_1O). One atom of chlorine can participate in the breakdown of up to 100 thousand molecules of ozone. In addition, direct release of chlorine from such substances as the cleaning solvent carbon tetrachloride destroys ozone, as do large quantities of dust released into the atmosphere from volcanoes. Chemicals that can damage the ozone layer are also found in animal feed and pesticides (methyl bromide) and even in typewriter correction fluid (methyl chloroform).

Tragically, we have known about and have been tracking the erosion of the ozone layer since the middle of the twentieth century. At that time, scientists from the British Antarctic Survey (BAS) noted that ozone levels above the Antarctic had dropped by 40 to 50 percent, but the information was not publicized until May of 1985 in an article published in the journal *Nature.* By 1987, half or more of the ozone in the upper atmosphere had been destroyed above the Antarctic in an area roughly the size of the United States. Not only is the hole big, but it is also as deep as Mount Everest is high (29,028 feet).

The hole is, in fact, so large that the ozone layer has been almost completely destroyed in the lower stratosphere above Antarctica. Approximately 95 percent of the damage done to the ozone layer is caused by chlorofluorocarbons (CFCs).

Discovered in 1928, CFCs can be produced inexpensively and are not flammable or smelly. These chemicals have been widely used as cooling agents in refrigerators, air conditioning units, freezers, and any other Freon-run appliances. The manufacture of the plastic or polystyrene foam used in packaging, insulation, and furniture stuffing releases large quantities of CFCs into the atmosphere. In the electronics industry, these chemicals are used to clean various computer parts because they do not damage the plastic.

Aerosol spray cans, introduced in the 1920s, once used CFCs as propellants. By 1974, an estimated 3 billion such cans were being produced annually in the United States. In 1978, the use of CFCs in those products was banned in the United States, Canada, Norway, and Sweden. Even with the ban, global production of CFCs had reached 700,000 tons by 1985.

In addition, chemicals known as halons occur in a number of fire extinguishers and contain bromine, which rises and attacks the ozone layer. Bromine is actually "more efficient" in destroying ozone in the stratosphere, but it is less abundant than chlorine.

Ramifications of a Depleted Ozone Layer

A 1 percent decrease in ozone levels can translate into a 3 percent increase in the amount of UV-B radiation reaching the Earth. This, in turn, translates into 10 to 15 thousand new cases of skin cancer. Scientists estimate that every 1 percent decrease in the ozone layer will result in a 3 percent increase in the incidence of basal cell and squamous cell skin cancer and an additional 50 thousand cases of cataracts each year. If the current rate of deterioration persists, there will be a 26 percent increase in skin cancer worldwide by the year 2000.

Addressing the Ozone Issue

Our overwhelming need to stop destroying the ozone layer is finally being addressed by the nations of the world. In 1987, twenty-three countries signed the Montreal Protocol, which called for a 50 percent decrease in CFC use by 1988. A subsequent protocol signed by sixty-four nations called for the elimination of all CFCs by the year 2000. Even with this action, it is estimated that an excess of 20 million tons of CFCs have already been released into the atmosphere. And CFCs are very stable; one type remains in the atmosphere for more than 130 years.

Now researchers believe the hole in the ozone layer above Antarctica will actually recover. They have already seen that by 1995, annual increases in certain prohibited halocarbons and fluorocarbons had declined, as had the levels of methylchloroform and carbon tetrachloride in the troposphere. Unfortunately, levels of other ozone-destroying gases in the troposphere continue to increase.

The noncompliance of some nations and individuals, as well as uncertainty about the amounts of CFCs and hydrochlorofluorocarbons (HCFCs) used in developing countries make it impossible to accurately predict when the ozone layer will be fully restored. Elicit trade in CFCs is also a problem. For instance, the use of Freon in automobile air conditioning has now been banned in the United States. People see this as an opportunity to make money by selling Freon on the black market (see "Black Market Threatens the Environment" on page 15). However, if the limitations that have been imposed on the use of CFCs and HCFCs are maintained, levels of ozone will increase as the concentrations of chlorine decrease. Some experts believe that these chlorine levels peaked near the beginning of 1994 and have now begun to decrease, but bromine from halocarbons was still increasing by mid-1995. Scientists continue to expect that the ozone layer will begin to recover by the turn of the century. This prediction is, however, dependent on widespread adherence to the restrictions in the international protocol. Without such adherence, the trend toward recovery could be delayed or even reversed.

And if you have any doubts that CFCs are behind the destruction of the ozone layer, scientists at the National Aeronautics and Space Administration (NASA) Langley Research Center in Hampton, Virginia, and at the University of California at Irvine conducted a four-year study that should put all doubts to rest. These scientists found that the rates of increase in the levels of chlorine and fluorine in the atmosphere closely matched levels near the Earth's surface. Various controls on the experiment assured that the increased levels of chemicals were not due to natural sources.

To assure that the ozone layer is fully restored, the World Resources Institute makes the following recommendations:

- Reduce CFC leakage.
- Increase CFC collection and recycling.
- Replace harmful CFCs with less damaging ones.
- Develop processes and products that do not use CFCs.

Adherence to the protocols by nations and to local ordinances by every individual is truly imperative. The ozone layer is essential to living things, affording protection from the ultraviolet light that can damage living cells.

INCREASING OUR EXPOSURE TO SUNLIGHT

It now appears that the ozone layer—nature's shield for the Earth—is more fragile than anyone could have imagined. It was not until technological advances of the twentieth century literally ripped a hole in the shield that most of us even became aware that the ozone layer existed. And if wanton destruction of that shield didn't pose enough danger to our health, changes in manners, morals, and lifestyles further increased our risk of skin cancer.

Black Market Threatens the Environment

Silk stockings are a thing of the past. Their demise was, no doubt, hastened during World War II when all available silk was being used to manufacture parachutes. Soldiers who bought silk stockings for their girlfriends were trading in the black market—buying goods in violation of restrictions such as price controls or rationing.

During World War II, black market operations were commonplace. Many items were in short supply because they were being used to support the war effort. In most of the nations at war, rationing and price fixing were instituted to ensure availability of scarce items. In the United States, black marketeers traded heavily in meat, sugar, tires, and gasoline, whereas in Great Britain, clothing and liquor were popular black-market items. After the war, Eastern European countries had meager industrialization and many consumer goods found their way to the black market. In Communist Russia, for instance, American-made blue jeans were bought and sold illegally.

The black market is still in existence but usually involves the exchange of foreign currency for domestic. This is a popular practice when official exchange values are too high in terms of the purchasing power of foreign money. Now, another product is worth more than its weight in gold on the black market.

CFC-12, also known as Freon, once the primary coolant for automobile air conditioners, has joined narcotics as the most lucrative contraband for smugglers. Law enforcers are hard pressed to stop them. In fact, six federal agencies in the

United States are attempting to shut down this black market in an effort called the "National CFC Enforcement Initiative."

Smuggling of CFCs, the chemical deemed responsible for the destruction of the ozone layer, is popular because the United States is phasing out production. The only available alternatives are far more expensive. Although the chemical is being phased out globally in accordance with a 1987 treaty, it is still available in some countries.

More than 80 million cars built before 1984 still use Freon in their air conditioning systems. Despite the knowledge that Freon contributes to the destruction of the ozone layer and an epidemic in skin cancer, car owners eagerly scoop up the contraband. These short-sighted individuals would do well to heed the words of the head of the Environmental Protection Agency: "CFC smugglers put the health of American families at risk."

Before the dawn of the industrial age, pale skin was considered a sign of the aristocracy—or at least of the well-mannered. A red or tanned complexion indicated that a person was "common." Ladies of fashion always carried parasols to protect them from sunlight. Furthermore, the morality of the times dictated that men and women wear long swimsuits that covered their bodies almost completely. Then in the 1920s, Coco Chanel, a French designer whose influence was enormous, popularized the suntan. Although she was a fashion maven, neither Chanel nor her followers considered the implications of traditional fashion. They, for instance, ignored the fact that desert dwellers such as the Bedouin tribes have always worn long flowing robes that protected them from the sun's rays.

The Hazards of Tanning

Currently, Americans spend an average of 1,600 hours in sunlight each year, and if natural sunlight isn't available, they head for tanning salons. Most people—including 80 percent of the tanning-salon operators interviewed in a recent survey—believe artificial light does not cause cancer. Sadly, they are all incorrect. In fact, Swedish studies conducted from 1988 to 1990 among 740 people concluded that melanoma patients had used sunbeds and sunlamps significantly more often than those who did not have skin cancer. Sunbeds and tanning salons make use of both UV-A and UV-B rays. UV-A rays can contribute to the formation of wrinkles and brown spots. *The Merck Manual* points out, "As many such light sources contain some UV-B, some long-term deleterious effects should be expected." Dr. Arthur Rhodes of the University of Pittsburgh School of Medicine contends that UV-A rays work with UV-B in causing skin cancer. The reference book *Drugs of Today* claims ". . . the ultraviolet part of the electromagnetic spectrum produced by the sun as light, in particular UV-B (320–290 nm), is responsible for producing long-term solar skin damage (keratosis) and skin cancers."

Increased UV-B is a particular problem in urban areas. High levels of nitrogen oxides from car exhausts react with sunlight to form photochemical smog that increases ozone in the troposphere. The ozone is formed when the nitrogen gas in sunlight mixes with hydrocarbons and nitrogen oxides. In the troposphere, ozone gas serves no protective function; it is, in fact, toxic at this level.

Physicians believe that exposure to UV-B is particularly risky for children. They feel that four to five periods of prolonged intense exposure before the age of sixteen can increase the risk of skin cancer. And the association between skin cancer and sunlight is not merely hypothetical; the evidence abounds.

Consider that between 1981 and 1991, the skin cancer rates

in Scotland doubled. During this same period, springtime levels of ozone over much of Europe decreased by 8 percent. Skin cancer affects fair-skinned, red-haired people in particular because they lack the melanin responsible for suntans that help to filter out harmful UV-B rays. No wonder that the increased rate of skin cancer in Scotland was blamed on the inhabitants' more intense exposure to sunlight. This exposure is no doubt equally responsible for the 7 percent yearly increase in the rate of skin cancer in Britain.

Since 1978, according to the Environmental Protection Agency (EPA), ozone over the United States has been depleted by 4 to 5 percent. It is not, then, surprising, that in 1995, approximately 400,000 cases of basal cell and squamous cell carcinoma were reported. Although these conditions are considered curable forms of skin cancer, approximately 1,900 deaths will occur as a result of such cases. Another 7,200 deaths will result from cases of malignant melanoma. In fact, EPA reports indicate that increased exposure to UV-B may cause 200 thousand skin-cancer-related deaths in the United States over the next fifty years. (More detailed information on the various forms of skin cancer is presented in Part Two.)

A FINAL WORD

People must now recognize the dangers of excessive exposure to the sun. Cancer issues aside, UV rays cause sunburn, which can be extremely painful. Unfortunately, avoiding excessive sun exposure can require radical alteration in lifestyle. If people find it so difficult to give up smoking and diets high in fat, how easy can it be for them to give up time outdoors? How likely are children to restrict their time in the sun—their time swimming, roller blading, playing ball—to protect themselves from a future possibility? Our time in the sun is so important to us that the rates of skin cancer continue to rise, presenting problems for which we must find solutions.

Part Two

The Problem—
Skin Cancer

*One would like to think that at least Mother
Nature would not place a carcinogenic burden
on the people of this planet.
   This, unfortunately, is not the case.*

Office of Technology Assessment
Cancer Risk

W e love the sun. It warms and comforts us. It bright-
ens our spirits. It helps plants grow. When the
summer sun shines, outdoor living becomes the
norm. We picnic, play, swim, even sleep in the sun.
And then, summer sun passes into gray skies of winter. Our
tans are gone, all but forgotten. But the damage remains: The
seeds of tomorrow's wrinkles and the roots of skin cancer have
been planted. And the tragedy is that we have brought it upon
ourselves—not only by worshipping the sun but by failing to
protect our environment and ourselves.

More and more often, scientists and physicians warn us of the dangers in too much exposure to the sun. And the statistics bear harsh witness to the truth of their words.

THE EPIDEMIC OF SKIN CANCER

According to a recent report in the *Medical Herald*, skin cancer is the most commonly diagnosed form of cancer in the United States. Researchers estimated that 1 million cases of skin cancer were diagnosed in 1997, and of these cases, 95 percent were squamous cell or basal cell carcinomas. Of the remaining cases, there were approximately 32,000 cases of melanoma—the most deadly type of skin cancer—with 6,800 of them ending in death.

Despite all the medical advances touted almost daily in the media, the death rate from melanoma *tripled* in the past four decades. Between 1973 and 1992, melanoma deaths increased 34 percent. At long last, the death rate from melanoma is declining, but no miracle cure lies behind the lower numbers. The American public's awakening sense of responsibility for its own health gets all the credit. The death rate has dropped only because Americans are seeking medical help more promptly, but the statistics still bode no good.

Melanoma rates are now increasing more rapidly than rates of any other malignancy. Just consider that the United States population increased 10 percent between 1980 and 1987 while the number of skin melanomas increased 83 percent! Approximately 30,000 Americans now have or have had melanoma. It is the most common cancer in women aged twenty-five to twenty-nine, and is second after breast cancer in women aged thirty to thirty-four.

What is the reason for this alarming increase in skin cancers? To fully understand the causes, we must first understand what skin cancer is.

UNDERSTANDING CANCER

Approximately 200 diseases are grouped together under the heading "cancer" because of the similarity in their growth patterns. All cancers are believed to originate from one "transformed" cell that does not respond to normal controls over cell growth. The offspring of this cell may grow and multiply, producing a tumor.

All tumors then—no matter where, no matter how big or how small—begin in one single cell. And the human body is made up of billions of cells, the smallest functioning unit of an organism. Each cell, as seen in Figure 2.1 on page 24, has a covering called a *cell membrane* that surrounds a fluid called *cytoplasm*. The membrane permits certain things to enter the cell while keeping others out. Inside the cell are compartments formed by membranes that branch off from the cell membrane and cytoplasm. There is also a nucleus, which directs the cell's activities. Inside this nucleus is DNA—deoxyribonucleic acid—which contains genetic information that is maintained in units called *genes*. These genes are strung like beads into chromosomes that contain DNA and protein. In addition to determining your features, genes transmit information to tell cells what chemicals to make, how much, and when.

Information is transmitted from the nucleus into the cytoplasm by RNA—ribonucleic acid—which is responsible for the transmission of genetic information and the synthesis of proteins, some of which are hormones while others are enzymes.

In the 1960s, scientists became aware that normal cells in all vertebrates carry genes whose abnormal expression can lead to cancer. Known as *protooncogenes*, these 3 to 4 thousand genes were discovered by Nobel Laureate Michael Bishop. Under certain circumstances, the protooncogenes become altered and are then known as *oncogenes*. These oncogenes can cause normal cells to transform into cancer cells.

In other words, we all carry genes that have the potential to

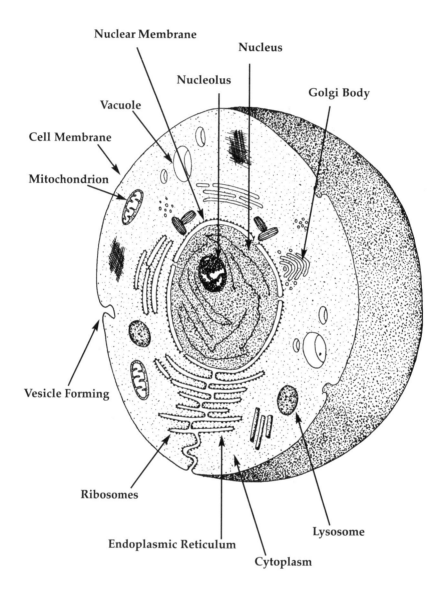

Figure 2.1.   A Living Cell

cause cancer, which occurs when something changes the DNA so that it activates oncogenes. Substances that can cause changes in DNA are called *carcinogens* and include various chemicals, radiation, and some viruses (hepatitis B, Epstein-Bar, HTLV, papilloma). These carcinogens may damage a weak point on a chromosome and prevent genetic controls from keeping the oncogene stable. This is sometimes called the *initiation phase* of cancer.

The change in DNA signals cells to grow and divide more rapidly than is normal. When a cell divides, each of its offspring receives a full set of genes, including the oncogenes. The cell replicates without control, producing millions of similar self-replicating cells. Soon, a growing mass of cells forms. As the mass grows, its cells may lose their unique characteristics and become "dedifferentiated." Parts of the resulting cell mass may directly invade adjacent tissue or may reach more distant parts of the body via the circulatory system.

Because cancer cells do not stick together in a mass as well as normal cells, single cells or groups can break away and be carried along the blood or lymph vessels. This is metastasis. The ability to spread or metastasize to other tissues characterizes a tumor as *malignant* or *cancerous*. Cell masses or tumors that remain in the tissues where they arise are classified as *benign* or *nonmalignant*. Eventually, a malignant mass will crowd out, starve, or choke normal cells that no longer have the nourishment or space they need. Cancer is a killer precisely because it destroys normal tissue and chokes off organs.

Cancers are characterized by the types of cells in which they arise. According to this classification system, there are three basic groupings:

1. Sarcoma
2. Leukemia and lymphoma
3. Carcinoma

A sarcoma is a malignant tumor that develops in connective tissue. In leukemia, white blood cells proliferate without control, which usually leads to anemia, impaired blood clotting, and enlargement of the lymph nodes, liver, and spleen. Lymphoma is cancer of the lymph nodes and other lymph tissues. Carcinomas are the most common cancers, accounting for 90 percent of cancer cases. They develop in the epithelial tissues that cover body cavities such as the lung, bowel, kidney, breast, and uterus. Carcinomas also develop in the skin or external epithelial tissue. In fact, the skin is the most common site in which carcinomas develop.

THE SKIN—YOUR LARGEST ORGAN

The skin is the largest human organ, measuring twenty square feet on an average male and seventeen square feet on an average female. The skin protects the body from various environmental factors such as heat and cold, as well as from trauma, toxins, and pollutants. Because the skin's outer layer is dry, the growth of bacteria is inhibited. The skin also plays a crucial role in the production, storage, and release of vitamin D, which is an essential component for the absorption of calcium and phosphorus.

The outer epithelial layer of the skin is called the *epidermis*. There are several layers to the epidermis. Cells from a lower layer called the *stratum basal* or *basal cell layer* move up to replace cells in the stratum corneum. Some believe that skin cells' ability to grow and reproduce on a regular basis may explain why skin cancer is so common an occurrence.

In the stratum spinosum, a central layer sometimes referred to as the *prickle cell layer*, there are Langerhans cells. These star-shaped cells are important components of the immune system, trapping invading organisms and aiding in their destruction. Langerhans cells, which are named for the German anatomist Paul Langerhans, can be damaged by ultraviolet radiation.

Some scientists, therefore, believe that a breakdown in the immune system contributes to the development of skin cancer.

The second layer of skin beneath the epidermis is referred to as the *dermis*. It contains blood and lymph vessels as well as nerves. Largely collagen, bundles of protein, and elastin fibers that can be stretched 100 percent and return to their original size, the dermis has a layer of fat under it. The dermis and underlying fat protect internal organs and bones.

At the junction of the dermis and epidermis are found melanocytes, cells that produce melanin, the substance that imparts color to skin and hair. Melanin normally shields skin from ultraviolet radiation. Melanocytes have branching processes that allow melanosomes to be transferred to the epidermis, causing pigmentation. The number of melanocytes is constant in people; it is the amount of melanin produced that gives each of us a unique complexion. Because melanin protects skin from damaging ultraviolet radiation, the darker your skin color, the lower your risk of skin cancer. However, during the process of tanning, the skin is injured, and repeated injury increases the risk of skin cancer. In fact, we now know that excessive exposure to sunlight—particularly blistering burns in young children—is a primary cause of cancer.

RECOGNIZING SKIN CANCER

As our awareness of the risks and dangers of skin cancer have increased, many of us have become concerned that various skin growths may be cancerous. Most are not, but some may be, and others may be precancerous.

Benign or Precancerous Skin Conditions

The overwhelming majority of skin conditions are completely benign. Some of these, such as skin tags and lipomas (soft fatty

The Skin Cancer Answer

nodules), may be treated for cosmetic reasons or because they are prone to irritation. Treatment is not, however, a medical necessity and may not be covered by insurance. The following conditions should, however, be checked by a health-care practitioner to ensure that any necessary treatment is initiated as quickly as possible.

Moles, Freckles, and Beauty Marks

Most moles, freckles, and beauty marks are groups of pigmented cells and pose no threat to health. These marks can be flat or raised, pink, tan, or brown. A mole, also called a *nevus* (the plural is *nevi*), is a risk factor because there is a *chance* it will become malignant. Furthermore, when clusters of malignant melanocytes develop, they may appear on the skin's surface as dark irregularly shaped moles.

Although most people are not born with moles, they will develop approximately forty by age twenty-five. These acquired nevi tend to flatten and disappear as we age. Congenital nevi, those that are present at birth, range in size from tiny to very large and have a higher risk of developing into melanoma. An irregular mole, also called a *dysplastic nevus,* is considered atypical. An atypical mole can be considered a precursor lesion because it *may* degenerate into melanoma. Atypical moles may appear on body parts that have been exposed to the sun, especially the trunk. They are less likely to be found on unexposed areas. These moles are larger than ¼ inch across with irregular or fuzzy edges. Tan to dark brown in color, they may have a pink background. Once a mole has begun to bleed and ulcerate, the cancer is considered incurable.

Lentigo Maligna

Lentigo maligna are flat marks that usually occur on the face and may have raised bumps inside. They are sometimes variegated in color, displaying shades of brown and black. Irregular in shape,

~ 28 ~

lentigo maligna may have the appearance of a stain. These marks commonly appear on elderly persons with light skin who have had lots of exposure to the sun. Approximately one third of lentigo malignas become malignant. Most physicians recommend that the lesions be excised before they become too large.

Keratoses

Keratoses or horny (callouslike) growths are another type of mark that appears on the skin. The most common are *actinic keratoses* (also called *solar* or *senile keratoses*) and *seborrheic keratoses*. Generally speaking, a keratosis occurs when a scaly layer is formed on the skin by an overgrowth of the epidermis. The condition begins with a small patch of dilated capillaries. A dry, rough, yellow or brown scale forms. If picked off, it may bleed. The lesion may become thick with a clear division from normal skin.

Actinic keratoses are characterized by thickening and inflammation of the skin and usually occur on the hands, face, neck, shoulders, and shins of middle-aged or elderly people. Sometimes these keratoses begin on the lip as a crack or an ulcer that doesn't heal and recurrently bleeds. Flat or elevated and rough in texture, the lesions can be an indication of excessive sun exposure. Sharply outlined and reddish or skin-colored, lesions of actinic keratosis may appear singly or in groups. A crust may appear that is later shed, revealing an ulcer. Although actinic keratoses grow very slowly, the rate of growth may increase if the lesions are irritated. If keratoses are not well established, they sometimes regress in the absence of sunlight.

Considered nonmalignant or premalignant, actinic keratoses have the potential to develop into cancer and the lesions are sometimes considered precancerous. Actinic keratoses are metastatic in less than 5 percent of the cases, but untreated they may lead to malignant squamous cell carcinoma (see page 31).

In fact, from 10 to 20 percent of patients with actinic keratoses will develop squamous cell carcinoma. During treatment of this skin growth, the lesions are biopsied and then curettage or cryotherapy is used. Topical application of the drug 5-fluor-ouracil (5-FU) is sometimes used when the lesion is widespread.

Seborrheic keratoses are benign, raised, yellow or brown, oval lesions with sharp margins. They often have a wartlike surface that is easily removed. These lesions may appear anywhere on the body except the palms and the soles of the feet. Cryotherapy is the conventional medical treatment of choice.

Keratoacanthoma

The benign lesion called *keratoacanthoma* must be examined by a physician and then under a microscope to differentiate it from a squamous cell carcinoma. Raised to 2 centimeters in diameter, this type of lesion has hard tissue at its center and is character-ized by rapid growth.

Leukoplakia

The premalignant condition known as leukoplakia occurs on oral or rectal mucosa or on the vulva as raised, whitish, single or multiple lesions. The condition is usually treated with cryother-apy or excision. To prevent recurrence, it is imperative that the irritant or predisposing factor such as chewing tobacco be elim-inated.

Cancerous Skin Conditions

Skin cancers are categorized as *melanomas, basal cell carcinomas,* and s*quamous cell carcinomas.* Kaposi's sarcoma (KS), which often affects AIDS patients, is also a form of skin cancer. The most common and curable types are squamous cell and basal cell carcinomas. Melanoma, the deadliest form of skin cancer, is so-named because it arises from the malignant transformation of melanocytes. For visual examples of these conditions, see Figure 2.2 on Color Plate One between pages 38 and 39.

Melanoma

Melanomas account for 2 percent of all malignancies, but the incidence is rising. This cancer is deadly and difficult to treat because it metastasizes quickly. Approximately 5 percent of the skin cancer cases are melanoma and 75 percent of the deaths associated with skin cancer are caused by melanoma. It is estimated that this cancer will kill 7,300 people this year. Rare prior to puberty, malignant melanoma afflicts white-skinned people twenty times more frequently than black-skinned people. Most likely to appear on the upper back and lower legs, this carcinoma sometimes occurs under nails and on mucous membranes. Research indicates that some families are genetically predisposed to developing melanoma.

The thickness of a melanoma lesion is often a factor in determining the prognosis. Lesions with a thickness of 0.75 millimeter have a cure rate of more than 90 percent. When lesions of 0.75 to 1.65 millimeters occur on the back, arms, neck, or scalp, the chance of metastasis is higher. At thicknesses of 4.0 millimeters, there is an 80 percent chance of distant metastases.

Squamous Cell Carcinoma

Squamous cell carcinoma (SCC) accounts for 20 percent of all skin cancers and is more likely to metastasize than basal cell carcinoma. Often secondary to chronic skin damage, SCC develops when underlying skin cells are damaged and a malignant tumor grows up from the layer of skin above the basal layer. Other predisposing conditions include actinic (solar) keratoses, xeroderma pigmentosa (a rare and often fatal disease characterized by scaly skin and extreme sensitivity to light), and leukoplakia.

SCC lesions resemble warts or ulcerations that do not heal. Rough, red, raised, scaly, and crusty, an SCC lesion is most likely to develop in fair-skinned people in areas that are exposed to the sun—the face, ears, neck, lower lip, nose, and the back of the hands.

Cases of SCC that begin from actinic keratoses have little likelihood of metastasizing (0.5 percent). Those arising from the penis, oral or rectal mucosa, vulva, and lips have a high rate of metastasis. Sunlight is the most common cause of SCC, but any carcinogen such as arsenic or radiation can precipitate development, and untreated actinic keratoses can give rise to malignant SCC. With sunlight, growth begins only after many years of exposure to UV-B rays. It is estimated that 3 percent of SCC cases caused by excessive sun exposure will metastasize. Sometimes SCC develops in scar tissue, skin ulcers, and tissue burned by x-rays. In these cases, there is a 20 percent chance of metastasis. A type known as *margolin's ulcer* arises in chronic wounds such as burns and osteomyelitis and is very aggressive.

More aggressive than basal cell carcinoma, squamous cell carcinoma may spread to structures beneath the skin. It is usually treated with excision, but Mohs' surgery (microscopically controlled excision) is used on lesions of the eyelids and ears and in the folds of the nose and lips. Radiation has a similar success rate but is reserved for inoperable lesions.

Basal Cell Carcinoma

Basal cell carcinoma (BCC) is the most common form of skin cancer, accounting for 75 percent of the cases and outnumbering squamous cell carcinoma cases four to one. Approximately 1,000 people in the United States die of BCC each year. BCC strikes men twice as often as women, and most cases appear on the sun-exposed skin of middle-aged or older people of Northern European ancestry.

This type of carcinoma occurs on the face, ears, neck, and head in 90 percent of the cases; the remaining cases occur on the trunk. BCC often begins as a small rounded lump with a pearly edge. There may be a few superficial transparent blood vessels. Frequently, BCC appears as an ulcer with a raw moist center. A hard border develops that may bleed. Scabs form continuously, fall off, and form again. This carcinoma occasionally appears as flat crusting or scaling lesions that are red or reddish gray. When irritated, these marks sometimes bleed.

BCC is caused primarily by UV-B radiation, but damage from other forms of radiation, arsenic exposure, burn scars, and vaccination marks are considered contributing factors. Although a malignant tumor that grows upward from the basal layer of cells, BCC is slow-growing and rarely metastasizes. It must be present for a long time before it will spread. Carcinomas of this type do, however, erode tissue so that left untreated, they may eventually kill. When removed, BCC has a tendency to recur in some places.

There are both sporadic and hereditary forms of BCC, which has four histologic types:

1. **Nodular.** The most common form, usually occurring on the head. These nodules are waxy or pearly in appearance.
2. **Sclerosing.** Yellow and waxy, usually found on the head and neck, with a high recurrence rate.
3. **Superficial.** Raised, pinkish, and scaling, these are usually found on the trunk and arms.
4. **Pigmented.** Dark brown or black, these lesions, which are often confused with melanoma, are relatively uncommon.

BCC lesions are usually treated with simple excision. When lesions are ill-defined or the disease is recurrent, Mohs' surgery is used as it is when the lesions are in aesthetically important areas. With conventional medical practice cure rates equal to surgery, radiation treatment is sometimes used when surgery is not possible. Following treatments, patients are checked every three months for one year and then biannually.

Be On the Lookout

It is recommended that you examine yourself monthly for any suspicious-looking growths or skin changes. (See "Monthly Self-Exam" on page 36.) If you notice any pigmented spots or growths on your skin especially if they change suddenly, be sure to consult your health-care practitioner. In addition, it is wise to undergo a yearly skin examination by your health-care provider. According to The Skin Cancer Foundation, knowing when to visit your doctor is as easy as A, B, C, D:

Asymmetry—one side of a skin mark doesn't match the other side.

Border irregularity—the edges of a skin mark are indistinct, ragged, or notched.

Color—various shades of tan, brown, and black appear in the mark. Specks of red, white, and blue give the mark a mottled appearance.

Diameter—a mark is at least the size of a pencil eraser (about 6 millimeters).

For clear visual examples of the ABCD's of skin cancer, see Figure 2.3 on Color Plate Two between pages 38 and 39.

As we have seen, early diagnosis is essential to the successful treatment of skin cancers. Knowing if you are in a high-risk group can help you determine whether your condition warrants medical attention. If you are in a high-risk group, you should be especially careful not to increase your risks.

RECOGNIZING THE RISK FACTORS

We have seen that carcinogenesis, development of cancer, begins with changes in deoxyribonucleic acid (DNA). What causes DNA to mutate or change? If we know the risk factors associated with skin cancer, perhaps we can protect ourselves.

Several factors that put us at risk have, in fact, been identified. They are: rate of cell division, inherited genetic defects, environmental factors, and some viruses. The Centers for Disease Control in Atlanta, Georgia, cites five risk factors for melanoma:

1. Light skin color.
2. A family history of the disease.
3. A personal history of the disease.
4. The presence of moles and freckles.
5. A history of severe sunburn early in life.

The CDC also lists four risk factors for both squamous and basal cell carcinoma. They are:

1. Chronic exposure to the sun.
2. A family history of skin cancer.
3. A personal history of skin cancer.
4. Light skin color.

Monthly Self-Examination

The best way to detect the early warning signs of skin cancer is to check your body thoroughly each month for suspicious growths or changes in moles (see the ABCD warning signs found on Color Plate Two between pages 38 and 39). Also, a yearly skin examination by a doctor is recommended.

1. With your arms raised in front of a full-length mirror, check the right and left sides of your body, including the underarms. ▶

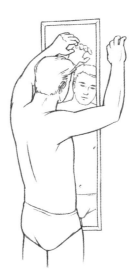

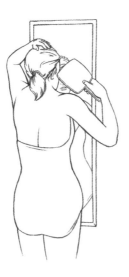

◀ **2.** Standing in front of the mirror, examine your head and face. Check the back of your neck and scalp with the help of a hand mirror. Use a blow dryer to lift the hair for a better look.

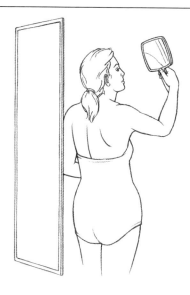

◄ 3. With your back to a full-length mirror, use a hand mirror to check your back, buttocks, and the back of your shoulders and upper arms.

4. Bend your elbows and examine the forearms, upper arms, and hands, including the palms and nails. ▶

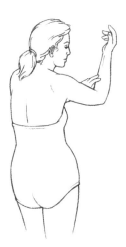

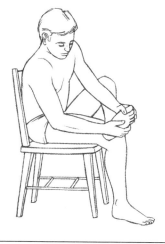

◄ 5. Sitting on a chair, check the back of your legs and feet, including the soles, heels, and spaces between the toes. Use a hand mirror to examine genitals.

Although we cannot control such risk factors as age, sex, rate of cell division, and genetics, being aware that we are in a high-risk group can help ensure an accurate diagnosis.

Rate of Cell Division

A particular cell's normal rate of division appears to be a risk factor for cancer. Some body cells are at greater risk of developing cancer than others. These cells appear at such sites as the skin, gastrointestinal tract, and bone marrow—places where cell division normally occurs throughout life. Cells in other organs such as the liver normally reproduce only to repair damaged tissue. There are even certain cells, such as nerve cells, that cannot multiply once they have reached maturity. Cancer of these cells does not occur in adults. It seems, then, that a cell's propensity to divide contributes to the overall cancer risk.

Genetic Factors

No matter what your lifestyle, your genes play a role in the development of skin cancer. Those with fair skin, light eyes and hair color, and a poor ability to tan are all at increased risk due to genetic influences. On the other hand, skin cancer is very rare among those with deeply pigmented skin.

Scientists now know that 10 percent of both UV-A and UV-B is blocked by the epidermis. The remainder of the rays can penetrate to deeper layers of the skin. UV-B activates melanocytes, which then produce melanin and a suntan. If a person has fair skin, there will be insufficient melanin to protect the skin and the person is likely to burn.

Squamous cell carcinoma has long been associated with excessive exposure to UV-B radiation. Now, researchers have

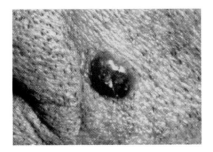
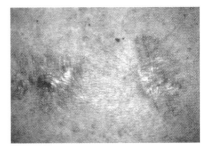

Basal Cell Carcinomas

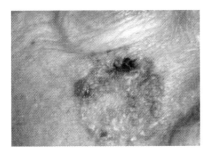
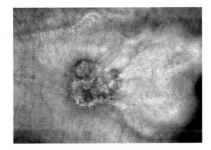

Squamous Cell Carcinomas

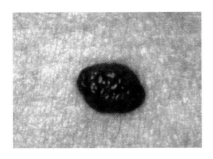
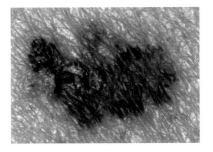

Melanomas

Figure 2.2. Examples of Cancerous Skin Conditions

The above photos are examples of cancerous skin conditions. A mark resembling one of the above photos is not necessarily cancerous. What is important is that you check with a qualified health-care provider upon discovering any unusual-looking skin mark.

* Photos courtesy of The Skin Cancer Foundation, Box 561, New York, NY 10156.

Color Plate One

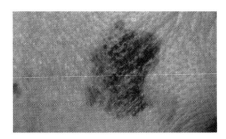

Assymetry

One side of a skin mark doesn't match the other.

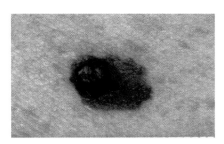

Border Irregularity

The edge of a skin mark is uneven, ragged, or notched.

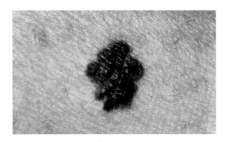

Color

Various shades of tan, brown, and black appear in the skin mark. Specks of red, blue, and white may give the skin a mottled appearance.

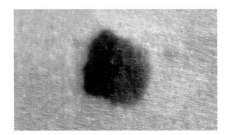

Diameter

A skin mark is at least the size of a pencil eraser (about 6 millimeters or $1/4$ inch in diameter).

Figure 2.3. The ABCD's of Detecting Skin Cancer

* Photos courtesy of The Skin Cancer Foundation, Box 561, New York, NY 10156.

Color Plate Two

discovered a very specific genetic change that is caused by UV-B. In squamous cancer cells, a change occurs in the DNA because of UV-B's action on a tumor suppressor gene.

Scientists have also identified the gene responsible for a rare inherited skin disease called *Gorlin's* or *basal cell nevus syndrome*. Those afflicted—approximately 1 in 100,000 people—have a predisposition to developmental abnormalities and a variety of cancers, especially basal cell carcinoma. The gene for Gorlin's is a version of a tumor suppressor gene called *Patched*. This gene is also mutated in some of the common basal cell carcinomas. The absence of this gene or its inactivation contributes to the uncontrolled development of cancer cells.

Two gene mappers from Stanford University in California found that *Patched* is situated on the long arm of chromosome 9. It lies near the presumed location of the gene for basal cell nevus syndrome. Researchers now believe that *Patched* plays a critical role in tumor suppression. If *Patched* doesn't function correctly, some genes may be abnormally active so that cells proliferate rather than differentiate.

In some cases, skin melanoma appears to be an inherited disease. One study followed eleven large extended families with melanoma and revealed that some families have a 50 percent higher risk of the disease. We know, too, that one in every ten melanoma patients has a relative with the disease. Again, an abnormal gene on chromosome 9 may be responsible for this predisposition to familial melanoma.

Genetics helps to explain why skin cancers can appear on areas of the body that are not exposed to the sun, such as the genitals and soles of the feet. In addition, some believe that having many large or irregularly shaped moles is an even more significant risk factor than exposure to the sun. Having five moles measuring at least ¼ inch has been associated with a ten-fold risk; the presence of a dozen such moles is associated with a forty-fold increased risk.

Environmental Risks

Because cells in the skin constantly reproduce and are often exposed to substances that can alter DNA, this organ has an especially high risk of developing cancer. In both human and animal studies, exposure to certain specific substances has been associated with cancer.

Many researchers believe that cancer is both multifactored and multistaged in its development. The first step occurs in response to an external stimulus and produces what is called a *latently pre-malignant cell*. There is no observable change in the cell or in its growth. If this cell is then exposed to another substance—a promoter—the cell becomes an "irreversible malignancy." Many years may pass between the initiation and promotion steps. Some substances act both as initiator and promoter; these are considered *complete carcinogens*.

The likelihood of cancer also seems to grow as a consequence of increased exposure to outside influences. More than half of all cancer occurs in cells that are in direct contact with the outside environment—again, the skin and linings of the gastrointestinal tract, as well as the lungs and cervix. This phenomenon is often cited in support of cancer as environmentally determined rather than a natural consequence of aging.

Among the first factors recognized as carcinogenic to humans were those that most affect the skin: ionizing radiation and ultraviolet light. These have been associated with some lip cancers and many squamous cell carcinomas, and they are considered the principal cause of basal cell carcinomas on the faces and necks of fair-skinned people.

Ionizing Radiation

Ionizing radiation occurs when high-energy radiation passes through a substance, causing the formation of ions—atoms that gain or lose electrons, thereby acquiring an electrical charge. Alpha and beta rays, as well as x-rays, are capable of causing ionization. X-rays' ability to penetrate makes them useful for radiography, radiology, and radiotherapy, but also makes the rays a potential carcinogen.

Ultraviolet Light

The sun emits three types of radiation: ultraviolet (UV), visible, and infrared. Along with infrared radiation, visible radiation provides light. It also penetrates the skin and warms us.

Light is actually a mixture of the seven colors of the rainbow—red, orange, yellow, green, blue, indigo, and violet—which always appear in the same order according to their wavelengths. Violet, at 0.0004 millimeters, is the first and shortest wavelength, and red, with a wavelength of 0.008 millimeters, is the longest. Rays of light just shorter than the red wavelengths are called *infrared rays* (*infra* is Latin for "below"). Other invisible rays lie beyond the violet end of the spectrum and are called *ultraviolet rays* (*ultra* is Latin for "beyond").

Both infrared and ultraviolet radiation are types of electromagnetic radiation, which is classified according to the length and frequency of its waves. Waves of UV or invisible radiation fall between visible light and x-rays on the spectrum. Seen in Figure 2.4 on page 42, the spectrum is the arrangement of light and other radiation according to wavelength, frequency, or other property. Measured in nanometers (nm) or billionths of a meter, invisible radiation has wavelengths that range from about 4 nm on the border of the x-ray region to about 380 nm, just beyond the violet in the visible spectrum. This UV or invisible radiation has many of the same properties as x-rays, microwaves, and gamma radiation.

Ultraviolet light, which amounts to less than 5 percent of the sun's radiation, has three different wave bands: UV-A, UV-B,

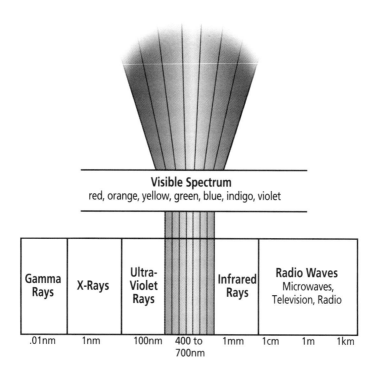

Figure 2.4. Electromagnetic Spectrum

and UV-C. The difference in the bands is determined by the length of the light waves. The range of light between about 320 and 380 nm is called UV-A, and the range from 280 to 320 nm is called UV-B. Only UV-A and UV-B rays—those longer than 290 nm—are able to reach the Earth's surface, and even these rays are largely absorbed by the ozone layer of the atmosphere. The shorter UV-C rays, which are considered particularly harmful to humans, are absorbed in the upper atmosphere or ozone layer.

Researchers once believed that UV-B rays, which are responsible for causing sunburn, were the only rays that damaged the skin. It had been believed that UV-A was less dangerous because it didn't seem to cause burns. It is now known that UV-A penetrates more deeply into the skin than UV-B, can cause skin cancer, and may suppress the immune system. According to Australian cancer researcher Dr. Bill E. Cham, "There are many types of skin cancers in humans. The most important environmental cause of those cancers in Australia, especially in Queensland, is exposure of susceptible people to the UV-B radiation of sunlight."

The evidence that UV radiation causes skin cancer is found among large groups of people who have high levels of exposure to sunlight. Hours of exposure to the sun, especially during childhood, is partially to blame for the increase in melanoma among the fair-skinned. People who have had severe blistering sunburns are twice as likely to develop skin cancer. Among adults, the risk is greatest for those who have intermittent intense exposure to sunlight. Skin cancers tend to occur in those who have indoor occupations but enjoy outside recreation. Perhaps because they are more likely to vacation in the tropics after having been indoors all year, wealthier people or people in the so-called "higher classes" are more likely to develop skin cancer than are laborers.

We know that the incidence of skin cancer in different countries correlates to the intensity of ultraviolet radiation. For instance, a survey in 1982 showed that there were 539 cases of skin cancer for every 100,000 people living in the Dallas-Fort Worth, Texas, area. The skin cancer rate in Iowa, on the other hand, was found to be 174 cases for every 100,000 people. We can safely assume that people living in the Dallas-Fort Worth area spend more time outside than do people in colder northern areas. In addition, people in Texas are exposed to more UV rays because these rays strike Texas more directly than they do in areas of higher latitudes, such as Iowa.

Consider, too, that in Israel, Orthodox Jews have a lower

incidence of melanoma than do nonreligious Israelis. The former always wear clothing that completely covers their bodies. And in Scotland, there has been a 300 percent increase in melanoma cases since 1970. Beginning in that year, the Scots steadily increased the time they spend on the beaches. Nowhere are the statistics more telling, however, than in Australia, where melanoma has reached epidemic proportions (see page 78).

No one really knows how UV causes cancer. Some hypothesize that it causes melanocytes, which normally divide at a slow rate, to increase rapidly. Rapid development causes a series of biochemical reactions that may lead to production of *growth factor*—biological chemicals that regulate cell growth. These chemicals may then initiate precancerous changes. Others believe that a melanocyte begins to change into melanoma when UV damages DNA and suppresses the immune system, limiting the body's ability to eliminate defective cells.

Tanning Agents

Recognizing the dangers of exposure to sunlight, many people try to tan without sun. All of the agents used to "bronze" the skin carry risks. Tanning beds cause your skin color to darken as the result of exposure to UV-A. Use of these beds may, therefore, be linked to melanoma. FDA scientists have concluded that people who use sunlamps about one hundred times in a year are increasing their exposure to melanoma-inducing radiation twenty-four times. The agency requires that these lamps have timers and controls that permit the user to turn them off. The labels must record the recommended distance from the sunlamp and include a warning about the dangers of their use. These lamps also must come with UV-blocking goggles.

People yearning to have a bronzed look also turn to tanning pills, which are taken internally. These usually contain carotenoid

The Sun—
Your Face's Worst Enemy

Basking in the sun feels so good and having a tan looks so terrific. But the sun is your face's worst enemy. Although ultraviolet radiation has been proven to cause skin cancer, some people's genetic makeup will prevent their getting the disease. But anyone who lives a long life will develop at least some wrinkles. The more time we spend in the sun, the more wrinkles we will develop.

The effects of UV-A are cumulative, eventually causing wrinkles and a loss of skin elasticity. According to a study reported in January 1996, UV radiation induces enzymes that degrade skin proteins such as collagen and elastin. Gary J. Fishers and a team of researchers at the University of Michigan Medical School believe that this process may be responsible for the type of skin aging that is caused by sunlight.

—a coloring additive that has not been approved by the FDA as a tanning agent and that may be harmful at high levels. The main ingredient in tanning agents is often canthaxanthin, which can deposit in your eyes as crystals and impair vision. Tanning accelerators that contain the amino acid tyrosine or tyrosine derivatives are not considered effective and may actually be dangerous.

Bronzers are cosmetics for external use; they simply stain the skin and can be washed off. Tan extenders interact with protein in the skin. The product color wears off over several days. The only FDA-approved color additive is dihydroxyacetone, which offers no protection against UV rays.

Other Risk Factors

Certain chemicals such as arsenic, and viruses such as Epstein-Bar and papilloma play a limited role in melanoma development. Although dietary factors have not been implicated, there is a possibility that a high-fat diet may be a risk factor.

A person's sex is also a risk factor with men being at greater risk than women. Between 1973 and 1992, the death rate for men with melanoma increased 48 percent. The Centers for Disease Control (CDC) in Atlanta, Georgia, calls this the largest sex-specific increase for any skin cancer. Interestingly, approximately 25 percent of those with malignant melanoma are women of childbearing age, and the risk appears to increase for women during pregnancy. Hormones that play a role in skin color circulate at increased levels during pregnancy. More than 10 percent of women in their first trimester experience changes in moles.

PREVENTING SKIN CANCER

Although we can do little at present to change our genetically determined risks for getting skin cancer, we can minimize our environmental risks. Even if our age, sex, skin type, and family medical history are stacked against us, we can still take measures to help ourselves.

Overwhelming evidence indicates that changes in diet can help prevent cancer. The higher your risk of developing cancer, the more important it is that you eat lots of fresh fruits and vegetables, and limit your intake of saturated fats. And we can certainly minimize our exposure to x-rays, making sure that this important diagnostic tool is used only when necessary and that protective lead aprons are used when appropriate.

Reducing our exposure to sunlight is yet another means of minimizing the risk of skin cancer. In fact, our first line of defense against skin cancer is protection from the sun; this is sometimes referred to as *primary prevention*. Early detection of skin cancers is considered the *secondary protection*. Both lines of defense require active participation on the part of the public, which must be educated about the hazards of sun exposure, ways of minimizing those hazards, and the early signs of skin cancer.

Prevention is considered so important that the Centers for Disease Control is currently developing a national program to target skin cancer prevention. In addition to developing and disseminating educational information aimed at children in particular, the CDC is seeking to evaluate the utility and value of the current UV index.

Understanding the UV Index

All summer long in fifty-eight cities in the United States, weathermen report the UV index in numbers ranging from 0 to 10. These numbers indicate the amount of UV rays that reach the Earth around noon. The higher the number, the greater is your exposure to UV rays, and the more likely you are to burn.

If the UV index is 0 to 2, you will burn in approximately sixty minutes at midday. If the index is 3 to 4, it will take you forty-five minutes to burn. You will burn in thirty minutes when the index is 5 to 6 and in fifteen to twenty-five minutes when the UV index is 7 to 9. Once the index reaches 10, which is routine in tropical climates, it takes only ten minutes to burn. If the index is 5, it's best to use a sunscreen with an SPF (sunscreen protection factor) of at least 15; if the UV index is 10, you'd better apply a product with an SPF of 30 and cover up. (Detailed information on sunscreens is presented beginning on page 48.)

The UV index is a joint effort of the National Weather Service, the Environmental Protection Agency, the Centers for Disease Control, and other health groups. UV forecasts cover a radius of about thirty miles for each of the cities included in the report. You can find out about your local UV index in the newspaper or on the Internet on the National Weather Service's Climate Prediction Center's home page at http://nic.fb4.noaa.gov.

To prevent the development of skin cancers, the CDC strongly recommends that people reduce or minimize their exposure to the sun and to UV radiation. Specifically, it suggests:

- Reduce direct exposure to the sun, especially between 1 P.M. and 4 P.M.
- When outdoors, especially on sunny days, wear a broad-brimmed hat and other protective clothing.
- Pay attention to the daily ultraviolet (UV) index, now available in fifty-eight cities.
- Avoid UV tanning beds.
- Use a factor 15 sunscreen (SPF 15) to help protect against ultraviolet A and B radiation.

Many people ignore every recommendation except for the last. They believe sunscreens alone provide sufficient protection. Wrong. Maybe dead wrong.

Sunscreens

Since the late 1970s, Americans have been spending more and more on sunscreens and sun-block products. The annual expenditure has now reached more than $525 million. Despite the increased use of sunscreens, skin cancer rates keep rising. In this same period, visits to physicians due to skin cancer have increased more than 50 percent. The FDA, researchers, and physicians are beginning to wonder whether sunscreens protect people against cancer or actually increase their risk.

First formulated in 1928, sunscreens then were made of iron oxide and petroleum jelly. As time marched on, the effectiveness of these sunscreens diminished. The fault lay not in the preparations as much as in the destruction of the ozone layer, which allowed increasing numbers of UV rays to reach the Earth.

Increasing use of sunscreens in an era of rising skin cancer rates led to FDA concern about confusing and possibly misleading claims. The FDA proposed various guidelines for the products in 1978, reviewed them in 1988, and revised them in 1993. In that year, the FDA issued a monograph regarding standards of safety and effectiveness. As a result, sunscreen labels must include statements about the sun's potential harm and the product's ability to protect people.

One of the earliest discoveries about sunscreens was that para-aminobenzoic acid or PABA, once a common ingredient in sunscreens because it absorbs UV rays, can cause allergic reactions in sensitive individuals. PABA in today's products has been replaced by salicylates, cinnamates, and avobenzone or Parsol 1789.

Today, there are two basic types of sunscreen—physical, which reflects and scatters UV rays, and chemical, which absorbs them. Physical sunscreens, which are often thick white creams, are not chemical-free; they contain either zinc oxide or titanium dioxide. Modern physical blockers are less sticky and unattractive than they had once been. The newest products do not leave a white film on your skin and are excellent protection against both UV-A and UV-B rays. They are water-resistant, but exposure to the sun may cause them to melt away, and they should be reapplied every two hours. Researchers now know that solid particle filters, sometimes called *micropigments*, do a fine job of blocking the sun by forming a protective layer on the skin. Some new formulas even include antioxidants.

Considered broad-spectrum, some of the latest chemical sunscreens absorb both UV-A and UV-B rays, and usually contain a

A Fig Leaf Won't Do It

Adam and Eve walked naked in the Garden of Eden. When they left the Garden, they donned fig leaves, not as protection against the elements but to hide their nakedness. Those of us who wish to hide our nakedness today will probably find fig leaves inadequate, unfashionable, and impractical.

If we put issues of morality aside, fig leaves just don't cut it as protective clothing. Because we are aware of the risks inherent in exposure to sunlight, we should be aware that clothing can be our best protection against UV radiation and our most complete protection against skin cancer.

Begin by being aware that fabrics differ in the UV protection they provide. Unbleached cotton absorbs UV while satiny polyesters and silk reflect it. Polyester crepe, viscose (a type of rayon), and bleached cotton permit UV to pass through to your skin. Tightly woven fabrics such as cotton twill keep out more light than broad weaves such as crepes or woven straw. Straw hats, then, are not your best protection, but a cotton hat with a three-inch brim all around would be optimal.

The color of the fabric also plays a role in protection against UV rays. White may make you feel cooler, but dark colors absorb more UV. And if you wear a T-shirt when you swim, remember that one-third of sun protection is lost when a fabric is wet.

Some companies today are manufacturing items of clothing that have SPF ratings. These garments are regulated by the FDA as "medical devices." Manufacturers include Sun Precautions (800–354–0203), which has a full line of sun-protective clothing for men, women, and children, and After the Stork (800–441–4775), a company that sells SunSkins—

children's clothing that blocks 50 percent more UV rays than regular clothing does.

And don't forget your eyes: UV exposure is a prime contributor to the development of cataracts. Sunglasses should be more than a fashion statement; they should block 99 to 100 percent of both UV-A and UV-B rays. If the label doesn't indicate that the glasses block these rays, do not buy them. Do try to buy the type that wraps around so that light does not get in at the sides.

So remember to dress for the occasion. On sunny days, don appropriate clothing, put on a hat, and wear your sunglasses!

physical blocker as well. Gavin Greenoak, scientific director of the Australian Photobiology Test Center, believes that these broad-spectrum sunscreens are the best products available. If the product you have purchased is a sunblock, it provides a physical barrier that causes UV to reflect and scatter off the skin. There are approximately twenty FDA-approved sunblocking agents that can protect you against UV-A. These include titanium dioxide and zinc oxide. Chemicals that can shield you from UV-B include cinnamates, patamates, and benzophenones.

Be sure to read the label of the product you are using. Benzophenone-3 and oxybenzone work well to block UV-B. Titanium dioxide is a natural mineral that blocks both UV-A and UV-B. Labels will also tell you if a product is water resistant, in which case it affords full protection for forty minutes in water and also provides protection even if you sweat heavily. You will get even more protection from a product that is labeled "waterproof." The FDA advises manufacturers to list the sunscreen protection factor (discussed on page 52), for both before and after water and sweat exposure, and a few manu-facturers are doing so.

Because a variety of factors determines the likelihood that you will burn, the use of sunscreens can be more important for some people than for others. For instance, those taking certain medi-cines may be more likely to experience the sun's harmful effects. Antibiotics, antidepressants, diuretics, and retinoic acid (found in many acne preparations) may make your skin more susceptible to sun damage. In addition, you must take into account such factors as altitude, ambient temperature, recent exposure to sun, pollu-tion, wind, and season. Your proximity to the equator and increased altitude increase the amount of UV to which you are exposed. For every 1,000 feet of increased altitude, you will be exposed to 4 to 5 percent more radiation.

Before using any sunscreen, test it on your skin to see if you are allergic or sensitive to it. Apply a small amount on the underside of your forearm and wait approximately twenty-four hours to see what happens. People with sensitive skin should avoid clear for-mulas, which often contain alcohol, and stick to lotions or creams. Clear formulas are, however, an excellent choice for those who have acne. These gel or water-based formulas are often noncome-dogenic, meaning they won't block your pores. Depending upon the conditions of your sun-exposure, you may need sunscreen that is waterproof, sweatproof, hypoallergenic, or fragrance-free (important if you need to avoid insects). Consumers should be aware that sunscreens do not have an indefinite shelf life; discard any remaining product after a year.

Sun Protection Factor (SPF)

No matter what their ingredients, today's sunscreens are rated by the FDA with what is known as an SPF—sun protection fac-tor. The higher the SPF number, the more protection you will get. This rating, however, can be misleading. Some sunscreens offer no protection against UV-B rays. Furthermore, SPF is a measure of protection from sunburn, *not* from cancer. Be aware, too, that products with an SPF greater than 30 aren't significantly more effective. In fact, the FDA claims the difference between SPF 30 and 40 is so small, it's nonexistent. The most important thing to understand about sunscreens is that *none of them is 100 percent effective.* You should certainly use them, but don't be lulled into a false sense of security. Whether you use sunscreens or not, regardless of your skin type, you *will* burn if you stay out in the sun long enough.

Be aware that the SPF number is not an indication of how many hours you can stay in the sun without burning. Rather, it indicates how much "longer than normal" you can stay in the sun without getting burned. Simply multiply the SPF number by the number of minutes it normally takes you to burn in the sun. For instance, if you normally burn in twenty minutes and you apply a sunscreen with an SPF of 15, you can stay in the sun for five hours without burning (20 minutes x 15 SPF = 300 minutes = 5 hours). And five hours is the maximum protection you will get; you will not get ten hours of protection if you reapply the product.

Although most people are aware that experts recommend using sunscreens with an SPF of at least 15, many forget to use them on hazy days. There is still a risk of sun exposure on these days because 85 percent of the UV rays can penetrate through clouds. People also forget that sunburn-producing rays can penetrate clear water to a depth of one foot; they neglect to apply sunscreen when swimming and often suffer severe sunburns.

In addition, few people are using adequate amounts of the sunscreen they buy. Liberal amounts—at least one ounce per person—should be applied fifteen to thirty minutes before going outside. Dermatologists disagree about the need to apply sunscreens a while before exposure to the sun. Some researchers claim that it takes thirty minutes for the chemical to achieve a good bond with the skin and recommend that sunscreens be applied from thirty to sixty minutes before you will be exposed to the sun. Of course, you don't have to lie on the beach to be exposed to UV; approximately 80 percent of your total exposure to the sun comes from doing everyday things like walking from your house or office to your car.

Remember to reapply your sunscreen every two hours and more often if you are active. And don't rub the product into your skin; it should sit on the surface. Don't forget to protect your lips, which have no melanin to protect them from UV. People with thinning hair should also apply sunscreen to their scalps, and we should all use it on our eyelids, being careful not to get any in the eyes. If sunscreen does get in your eyes, rinse them with water. Don't use sunscreens on infants younger than six months; their skin may not be able to handle the chemicals. Children from six months to two years of age should use a sunscreen with an SPF of at least 4.

A False Sense of Security

Using sunscreens may be giving people a false sense of security. Robin Marks, a dermatologist in Melbourne, Australia, worries about people constantly applying large amounts of chemicals to their skin. He's not sure that the long-term effects won't turn out to be carcinogenic or have some genetic effect on people's offspring.

Furthermore, some researchers now believe that infrared light—the sun's heat—may actually boost the damaging action of UV-B. Since sunscreens have no effect on infrared light, they may not adequately protect you from skin cancer. More frightening still are the claims that exposure to ultraviolet light may impair the immune system's ability to fight melanoma. Although sunscreens may protect against sunburn, they may not protect against these other effects.

For Sunburn Woes

Sunburn is characterized by redness, tenderness or pain, swelling, and blistering. To relieve the discomfort associated with sunburn, the American Academy of Dermatology recommends that you apply wet compresses or take cool baths. You can also use over-the-counter hydrocortisone creams and various moisturizers. More serious cases of sunburn involve fever, chills, upset stomach, and confusion. For these cases, you should consult a health-care practitioner.

Researchers at the University of Texas M.D. Anderson Cancer Center in Houston discovered an astonishing fact in studies with mice. Mice to whom sunscreen had been applied were exposed to UV-B rays for twenty to twenty-seven minutes twice a week for three weeks. A control group of "untreated" mice was similarly exposed. Both groups were also injected with melanoma cells. Researchers found that the radiation actually stimulated growth of the melanoma cells in *both* groups. Other studies have failed to show a decreased risk of melanoma with sunscreen use. While sunscreens may provide protection against basal cell and squamous cell carcinoma, there is no clear evidence that the products protect against malignant melanoma. In fact, some evidence indicates that the incidence of melanoma is actually higher among those who use sunscreens. People who use sunscreen may be spending more time in the sun and actually increasing their cancer risk.

Several studies indicate that sunscreens may not be effective against skin cancer. In two out of four studies of squamous cell carcinoma, sunscreens were *not* effective in protecting against the disease. Two studies of basal cell carcinoma revealed that people who use sunscreen were *more likely* to develop the condition. When the results of ten melanoma studies were reviewed, researchers reported that in five studies, people who used sunscreen were *more likely* to develop melanoma. In three of ten studies, no association was seen between sunscreen use and melanoma. In two of the ten studies, people who used sunscreens did appear to be protected against melanoma.

Adriane Fugh-Berman, M.D., medical advisor to the National Women's Health Network and medical director of the Taoist Health Institute in Washington, D.C., says, "While sunscreen clearly prevents sunburn, its effect on skin cancer risk is much murkier." Furthermore, Dr. Fugh-Berman contends that alternating exposure to UV-B and UV-A rays with exposure to UV-A alone may increase the carcinogenic effect of ultraviolet radiation. If you do not reapply sunscreen or you use it irregularly, you are alternating your pattern of exposure.

Cedric and Frank Garland, epidemiologists at the University of California at San Diego, point out that by blocking UV-B, sunscreens block the body's normal synthesis of vitamin D. This important nutrient helps regulate calcium and phosphorus levels and is vital to bone health. In one study, constant use of sunscreens was shown to decrease levels of vitamin D. This can be a significant problem since Americans get about 75 percent of their vitamin D from sunshine. The epidemiologists also believe that vitamin D may actually play a role in preventing melanoma.

Words of Caution

Remember, use of sunscreens does not make your skin impervious to the sun; there is no substitute for safe sun habits. Wearing protective clothing and staying indoors during peak sunlight hours are considered "effective" weapons against skin cancer. In fact, staying out of the sun is the only *sure* way to reduce your risk.

The Skin Cancer Foundation does, however, have a few other recommendations. The Foundation reminds us, for instance, that dark colors protect the skin from radiation better than light colors. When clothing is wet, it becomes transparent and offers less protection. Beware, too, of hazy days. In this weather, UV light is scattered in all directions by the water droplets in the air, thus increasing the risk of sunburns.

Increasing Public Awareness

Unfortunately, a recent survey conducted by the American Academy of Dermatology revealed that people who are at the highest risk for melanoma are least aware of its potentially lethal effects. Conducted in 1996, the survey revealed that approximately 42 percent of the respondents were unaware that melanoma is a form of skin cancer. This figure rose to 72 percent for those aged eighteen to twenty-four—ages at which the risks associated with severe sunburn are higher than in later life. However, approximately 80 percent of a person's lifetime sun exposure occurs before the person is eighteen years old.

Because of the survey and because it is critically important that parents be well educated so that vulnerable children will be protected, the CDC has launched a major campaign to raise public awareness through education about skin cancer.

TREATING SKIN CANCER

Despite repeated warnings about the need to avoid excessive exposure to the sun, the rate of skin cancer has increased dramatically. Measures are being taken to control the spread of the disease, but treatment of existing conditions remains a primary concern. Fortunately, skin cancer patients today have many treatment options: surgery, radiation, chemotherapy, or experimental therapies such as immunotherapy.

Successful treatment of skin cancer depends on attacking the disease in the early stages. Even melanoma is easy to detect and can be cured if treated early enough. If a carcinogen causes melanocytes to mutate and develop rapidly, a growth may appear. So long as this growth stays on the epidermis, the condition is not cancerous. If a melanoma begins to grow outward from the center, it can be surgically removed. If this melanoma remains, it may grow down into the skin and metastasis may then occur.

Current treatment methods for skin cancer include radiotherapy, a number of dermatological procedures, surgery, and chemotherapy. A number of natural treatments are also being used. Shark cartilage in a cream formulation is a relatively new and effective treatment option especially against Kaposi's sarcoma, and it has no negative side effects. One natural treatment that is derived from plant extracts of the genus *Solanum* has been found to be most effective. This particular treatment—a cream containing glycoalkaloids—will be discussed in detail in Part Three. The following section provides an in-depth look at each of the other treatment methods, all of which have a host of problems associated with them.

Radiotherapy

Prior to 1950, radiotherapy was used rather frequently to treat all forms of skin cancer. Radiation is sometimes effective as a cancer therapy because high-energy x-rays inhibit a cell's ability to grow and divide. Relatively large doses of radiation can, however, damage or kill the cells in normal tissue. The beam of radiation must be focused accurately enough to hit only tumor tissue. As Dr. Alvin Silverstein says in his book *Cancer: Can It Be*

Stopped?, "The big problem is to find ways to kill the tumor without killing the patient, too."

Radiation treatment often results in scar tissue that has no pigment and creates an indentation in surrounding skin. Such tissue may degenerate and actually undergo malignant changes.

Today, radiation is used to treat skin cancer when tissue removal would impair function, as on an eyelid, or cause excessive cosmetic damage. Sometimes a small amount of a radioisotope is inserted into the cancerous growth or a patient can swallow or be injected with radioisotopes. (Most of us are familiar with the radioactive-iodine "cocktail" that is used to diagnose and treat thyroid cancer.) In a case of inoperable metastatic melanoma, radiation may be used to provide symptomatic relief, such as the reduction of swelling and pain.

Dermatological Procedures

Certain procedures used to treat superficial cancers are less invasive than general surgery and are usually performed in a doctor's office. Referred to as *dermatological procedures*, these treatments—cryotherapy, curettage, diathermy, laser surgery, hyperthermia, and Moh's chemosurgery—all result in the formation of scar tissue, the lack of regrowth of normal tissue, and/or a high rate of cancer recurrence.

Let's take a closer look at these dermatological procedures to learn their benefits as well as their drawbacks.

Cryotherapy

Possibly the most widely used method of treating superficial skin cancers, cryotherapy (also called *cryosurgery*) uses extreme cold to destroy cancerous tissues. A probe equipped with a channel containing liquid nitrogen is applied to the lesions. Although we usually think of nitrogen as a gas, at -320°F it becomes liquid. Tissues with which the probe comes in contact freeze almost instantaneously. The treatment is not without its disadvantages. When the lesion thaws, patients experience pain, the subsequent formation of blisters, and eventual scarring.

Curettage

In this skin cancer treatment method, a curette—a sharpened spoon- or scoop-shaped surgical instrument—is used to literally scoop or scrape out the tumor. Bleeding is stopped through cauterization, often brought about with an electric current.

Diathermy

High-frequency electromagnetic radiation destroys tissue during diathermy treatment. The tissue is heated because of its resistance to the passage of the energy. When using this treatment method, it is, of course, difficult to control the radiation to ensure that only cancerous tissue is destroyed.

Hyperthermia

During hyperthermia treatment, the patient's blood is heated to between 106.7°F and 122°F with ultrasound or magnetic induction. Because blood circulation in tumors is relatively poor, the heat kills the tumors while blood flow in normal tissue dissipates the heat.

Laser Surgery

Laser surgery is frequently used to treat melanoma. During laser surgery, tissue is "cut" with a tightly focused beam of light having immense heat. Pigmented or colored melanoma tumors absorb more of the laser light than do the normal cells. In this case, laser surgery destroys only the cancer and not the normal tissues. Sometimes, dyes can be used to color cancer cells so that the same effect can be achieved. It is absolutely necessary that the aiming beam and the light beam be aligned prior to the procedure.

Moh's Chemosurgery

This skin cancer treatment is defined as "microscopically controlled excision after the tissue has been killed and hardened (fixed) with such chemicals as zinc chloride." During this procedure, successive layers of skin are shaved off and then examined until no cancer cells are found.

An ointment preparation of 5-fluorouracil (5-FU)—an antimetabolite that inhibits RNA and protein synthesis—is sometimes used as the fixative. Because it is not specific for cancer cells, 5-FU can damage healthy tissue. Therefore, considerable care and medical supervision are required during application of the ointment.

Skin Cancer Surgery

Various types of lesions that are not superficial can be treated only with more invasive methods such as surgery or chemotherapy. Surgery is the oldest form of cancer treatment. Indeed, Egyptian doctors were treating cancer with surgery 3,500 years ago (see "Ancient Surgery" on page 63). Currently, surgical therapy cures more cancer patients than does any other treatment.

Although conventional "under-the-knife" surgical procedures can more completely remove affected tissue than other techniques, these procedures do have disadvantages. If the lesion is large enough, skin grafting—putting healthy skin patches on areas denuded of skin—may be necessary, or reconstructive plastic surgery may be needed. In the attempt to get all the cancer cells, surgeons may have to remove some normal tissue as well as cancerous lesions. Scarring and, therefore, some amount of disfigurement are very likely to occur. In addition, there is a chance that the cancer will return.

A primary melanoma is usually removed surgically with local anesthesia as an out-patient procedure. A metastatic melanoma is usually removed in a hospital operating room with general anesthesia, and the patient can expect a substantial stay in the hospital.

Removal of a simple lesion can cost as little as $250. But the cost of curing a widespread skin cancer and bringing life back to normal is literally thousands upon thousands of dollars. Of course, medical insurance will cover most if not all of these costs. Many people, therefore, are unperturbed by the charges. They do not realize that they are actually paying exorbitant costs incurred by hundreds of thousands of cancer patients. Insurance companies charge each and every insured person a part of the total expenditure for medical care. Insured people do indeed pay for surgery, medicine, and doctors' time, but they pay the insurance company instead of the hospital, pharmacy, or doctor.

Removal of cancerous tissue can cause either minor or truly disfiguring cosmetic problems. There have, for instance, been cases of skin cancer in which the entire nose had to be removed. The popular fashion magazine *Mademoiselle* recently reported the case of a twenty-eight-year-old lawyer in Manhattan whose skin cancer surgery had serious side effects. The young woman had been diagnosed with a malignant melanoma on her lower right leg. A plastic surgeon removed the melanoma and the

Ancient Surgery

Surgery, often regarded as a life-saving technique, may actually have begun as a death technique. The ancient Egyptians, regarded as fine surgeons, probably gained their knowledge from the practice of embalming. Believing that a dead person's spirit would die if the body rotted, the Egyptians sought means to preserve the flesh. An involved cleansing, stuffing, and wrapping ritual preserved the body and began with removal of internal organs, which were preserved and stored in jars.

But the Egyptians were not the only ancients who knew about surgery. In India around 700 B.C., the Ayurveda was written. A comprehensive medical text, the Ayurveda describes a variety of surgical instruments. Indian physicians apparently performed many operations on the stomach and bladder and could even remove cataracts. Their skills as plastic surgeons were notable as they frequently rebuilt wounded parts of the body. For instance, Indian surgeons used hair to stitch up torn lips.

Ancient China also made notable contributions to surgery. The Chinese were the first to develop a technique to relieve the pain of surgery. The technique was a form of acupuncture, a procedure that is only now receiving the respect of the Western medical community.

surrounding tissue in a procedure that required forty stitches and left a three-inch scar. According to the lawyer, she "was awake during the surgery and could hear the skin being torn and removed. It was truly awful."

Surgical Risks

Surgical procedures—whether in- or out-patient—always involve the risks of infection, bleeding, and problems associated with the use of anesthesia. No matter how skilled the surgeon, how prestigious the hospital, risk exists.

Surgery always involves creation of a wound, and all wounds carry the risk of infection because the skin's function as a protective barrier has been violated. Even with a "clean" operation—one in which there is no infection and no involvement of the respiratory, urinary, or intestinal tracts—there is a 1 to 2 percent chance of postoperative infection.

According to the *Textbook of Surgery*, infection is a major source of disease and even of death in surgical patients. Factors associated with increased risk of infection include extremes of age, obesity, malnutrition, diabetes mellitus, acute or chronic steroid therapy, use of immunosuppressive drugs, a remote previously existing infection, presence of cancer, and irradiated tissue.

The rates of post-surgical infection depend on the type of operation, with the most severe risk occurring when the surgery involves tissue that is already infected, as in a case of gangrene. However, the risk of infection with any skin surgery is from 1.5 to 5 percent. The patient is the primary source of operative contamination and the operating team is the second source. As you can see, the protocol of scrubbing is neither ritualistic nor for show. Members of the operating team should scrub with an antiseptic for three to five minutes. But even this is not enough. Gloves offer the patient further protection from the possibility that members of the operating team may transfer infection.

Fever is considered a common postoperative occurrence. Although these fevers do not necessarily indicate the presence of infection, all wounds must be examined when fever occurs soon after surgery. Soft tissue infections with *Clostridia* or group

A *Streptococcus* spread rapidly and have high mortality rates unless treatment is initiated promptly. Fevers that occur by the third day after surgery are very likely to be caused by infection. Infections of the wound proper are usually not seen until the third through fifth day post-op.

Sometimes antibiotics are used prophylactically (as a preventive measure) before surgery to prevent wound infections. This is not, however, considered a substitute for good surgical technique. Antibiotics are, of course, used to treat infections that occur postoperatively. Such treatment carries its own risks, including rashes, allergic reactions, gastrointestinal symptoms, and the emergence of resistant strains, as well as superinfection with those organisms that are already resistant.

Other frequent postoperative complications include pain, bleeding, and croup. Far less frequent, but still a surgical risk, is death of the patient. Various factors are associated with an increased risk of death. These include:

- Age over seventy
- Compromised physical status
- Emergency as opposed to elective surgery
- Extensive procedure
- Associated illnesses

Some people who undergo surgery are at risk for cardiac complications. Conditions such as advanced age, myocardial infarct within six months, poor medical condition, elevated levels of the enzyme transaminase, and chronic liver disease increase the risk of cardiac complications. Those who have long been bedridden are also at risk.

Numerous risks are associated with the use of general anesthesia, which is required during any extensive surgical procedure. The chapter on anesthesia in the *Textbook of Surgery*, points out that in about half of major anesthetic catastrophes, human error constitutes a significant component of the problem. Recognition of this situation has led to increased training for anesthesiologists, including the use of simulators.

Although life-threatening complications from anesthesia are rare, it is not unusual to see such complications as headache, nausea, and vomiting, and slow emergence from the drug. Patients frequently experience a sore throat from intubation (insertion of a tube into the respiratory tract). In some cases, intubation may interfere with wound closure.

Respiratory complications are still another possibility. These are, of course, most likely to occur in those with pre-existing lung conditions. These complications also occur in patients with normal lungs who develop respiratory abnormalities as a result of anesthetic agents or the surgical procedure itself. This risk is increased during thoracic and upper abdominal surgery, and during operations lasting longer than three hours. The risk is also greater for those who smoke, are older than sixty, are obese, and/or are malnourished.

Though uncommon, neurological complications are considered a "vital concern" to the anesthesiologist and the surgeon. The physicians must exercise extreme diligence in the maintenance of appropriate oxygenation and circulation so that cerebral function is not impaired. Furthermore, pulmonary aspiration is a tragic surgical complication, which can be easily prevented if the patient's stomach is evacuated before general anesthesia is administered.

After receiving anesthesia, a patient must be closely monitored to ensure the proper volume of fluids and prevent a serious drop in blood pressure. Maintenance of the necessary volume of fluids requires careful and continual examination of the patient, including assessment of vital signs and urinary output. Even if this requirement is attended to with utmost diligence, there are cases in which it is difficult to estimate fluid requirements for the twenty-four hours following surgery.

Of course, these complications are all associated with major surgery performed under general anesthesia in an operating theater. But what of the procedures that are performed in a doctor's office with local anesthetics? Are these procedures without risk? Not at all. Any procedure that involves injury to living tissue necessitates healing. But healing is a complex process and the more cells and systems that are involved, the greater the chance that something can go wrong.

The most obvious side effect of surgery is scarring. Wound healing is complex, involving cellular and physiologic processes. Almost always, the healing of injured tissues involves scar formation—a cellular response in which necrotic tissue is replaced with scar tissue.

Approximately three days after any injury, including surgery, fibroblasts—cells that develop into connective tissue—appear and capillaries proliferate. These fibroblasts migrate into the wound and synthesize collagen fibers in bundles that enlarge and produce a dense collagenous structure or scar. Scar tissue on skin has the disadvantage of lacking sweat glands and hair follicles.

The scarring process is easily compromised in people who have poor nutrition. In fact, in animal studies, it has been demonstrated that wounds heal more slowly when protein is depleted. Deficiencies of vitamin C and vitamin A have been implicated in delayed wound healing. Some experiments have shown that supplements of vitamin A can ward off wound defects caused by radiation. Zinc is also considered important for the creation of new epithelial tissue. The lack of oxygen that occurs in poorly vascularized areas also causes delayed wound healing and may, therefore, be a risk factor for those with anemia.

Ensuring Healing of Wounds

Certain drugs or therapies should not be used prior to surgery. Preparations of shark cartilage, for instance, should not be used approximately two weeks prior to or following an operation because they impede the development of new blood vessels required in healing. One of the most serious impediments to wound healing is the use of steroids, which delays the rate of protein synthesis and inhibits normal inflammatory response.

In wounds, the inflammatory phase initiates the healing process. Within hours of the injury, the wound is filled with white and red cells, plasma proteins, and fibrin strands that are responsible for inflammation. Large doses of steroids inhibit the development of epithelial tissues as well as new blood vessels.

Where skin has been irradiated, wound healing is delayed. Although antimetabolic chemotherapeutic agents normally pose no impediment to wound healing, it is recommended that 5-fluorouracil (5-FU) be used with caution following major surgery. In addition, Adriamycin will decrease the rate of healing.

If wounds are to heal successfully, they must be cared for properly. Contaminated, devitalized, or dead tissue must be removed from wounds and accumulation of fluid must be prevented. In addition, exposed tissues cannot be permitted to dry. If they do, surface cells can die and blood flow in small vessels can be altered. Excessively tight stitches can restrict or obstruct blood flow at the edges of wounds. Permanent sutures can be the point of origin of an infection, and stitches that are present for a long time period can injure the skin and cause increased scarring. For this reason, when cosmetic considerations are important, sutures are removed earlier rather than later.

During the healing process, it is normal for wounds to contract. This wound contraction can have negative side effects. When large wounds contract in areas of the body involved in movement, there can be some degree of functional impairment.

The total time required for wound healing can be as long as one year after injury. During this period, the wound is said to be "remodeling," a process that involves changes in both color and size. Because the process can take so long, physicians often recommend that reconstruction or cosmetic procedures be delayed until remodeling is completed. This can pose significant problems for those whose injuries are cosmetically debilitating.

In any event, approximately 75 percent of skin cancer patients with advanced disease have multiple tumor sites, and surgery will probably not be helpful to them. These patients can, however, avail themselves of other treatment options such as radiation and chemotherapy.

Chemotherapy

Chemotherapy—predated by both surgery and radiation—is a relative newcomer to the field of cancer treatment. A variety of chemotherapeutic agents are in use today, including cytotoxic drugs—those that poison cells—hormonal agents, and immunologic drugs.

A Brief History

German scientist Paul Ehrlich, winner of the Nobel Prize in Physiology and Medicine, is often considered the father of chemotherapy. Late in the nineteenth century, he investigated the possibility that chemical agents might be useful in curing disease. He tested the usefulness of such substances in the treatment of infectious diseases by administering them to animals. In 1910, Dr. Ehrlich's experiments with arsenic compounds proved successful; his 606th compound—Salvarsan—was effective against the *Spirocheta pallida*, the organism that causes syphilis.

In the early 1900s, American physician George Clowes tested cancer-fighting chemicals in animals that had been implanted with cancer. Then, in December 1943, a United States navy vessel sank, causing an explosion of the mustard gas it carried.

Autopsies of sailors who had died from exposure to the poison revealed that the gas seemed to inhibit growth of malignant white blood cells. Soon nitrogen-mustard compounds, termed *alkylating agents*, were being tested in patients with Hodgkins and other lymphomas at the Yale-New Haven Medical Center.

Originally administered intravenously, nitrogen-mustard compounds were found to cause severe nausea and vomiting. However, the compounds did kill rapidly growing cells, especially lymphoma cells. Experiments confirmed that the toxic chemicals in mustard gas could be used to fight leukemia and lymph system cancers. So began the age of cancer chemotherapy.

Chemotherapeutic or cytotoxic compounds were actively sought from 1943 to 1975. In 1949 alone, 5,031 substances including organic and biological products, heavy metals, and dies were tested. Most showed no anticancer activity. Between 1955 and 1975, more than 400,000 compounds were tested against cancer. During that period, the National Cancer Institute (NCI) used 40,000 different compounds in conducting tests on just one form of mouse leukemia.

In the 1950s, childhood tuberculosis was successfully treated with a combination of compounds. Using several drugs in combination prevented the development of resistant organisms. Combination chemotherapy was next used to treat childhood leukemia. Researchers found that one agent, Aminoprerin, caused dramatic but temporary remission. Subsequently, several antileukemic agents were administered, followed by a year of maintenance therapy with one or two drugs. This therapeutic technique led to prolonged life and, in many cases, cures.

By the 1970s, chemotherapy was widely used. Clinical trials at this time focused on alkylating agents related to the nitrogen-mustard compound first used in the early 1940s. Scientists now know that these agents work by interfering with RNA transcription, which leads to cell death. In addition, antimetabolites (substances that compete with or replace a particular product of metabolism), natural products from plants, and various hormones were tested.

Antimetabolites interfere with the synthesis of DNA, RNA, and proteins, and prevent cell division. These drugs include 5-fluorouracil (5-FU), which is used for treating actinic or solar keratoses and superficial BCCs, as well as solid tumors in the breast, colon, and rectum. Drugs containing platinum are also used in the treatment of cancer. These drugs, which include cis-platin palladium, prevent replication of DNA by binding to it.

A current trend in chemotherapy is hormonal manipulation. With this kind of therapy, various hormones or their antagonists are administered, or hormone-secreting organs such as ovaries or testes are surgically removed. In 1896, surgeon George Thomas Beatson of Glasgow, Scotland, was the first to remove ovaries from premenopausal breast cancer patients. He believed that without the ovary's internal secretion, the tumor would atrophy. In 1904, J.W. White of Philadelphia demonstrated that castration of dogs led to shrinking of the prostate gland.

Some hormones used to treat cancer fall into the category of alkylating agents. Such agents make it difficult for DNA to produce the RNA that carries messages, thus preventing DNA replication. Alkylating agents such as the nitrogen-mustard compound first used in the 1940s (see pages 69–70) bind to DNA and proteins to inhibit cell growth. Other agents usually interfere with various stages of mitosis.

Use of immunologic drugs for the treatment of cancer is also referred to as immunotherapy, biologic therapy, or application of biologic-response modifiers. Immunologic drugs work either by manipulating the body's immune response or by improving a person's response to cytotoxic agents or radiation therapy by enhancing the function of bone marrow or blood cells. The much-touted drug interferon belongs to this class of drugs.

The immunologic agent dinitrochlorobenzene (DNCB) has brought about regression of skin malignancies. In addition, certain bacteria (e.g. attenuated tubercle bacilli [BCG]) have been used experimentally to treat melanoma. According to *The Merck Manual*, "Direct injection of BCG into melanoma nodules almost always leads to regression of the injected nodules, and occasionally of distant noninjected nodules."

The Trouble With Chemotherapy

Chemotherapy is not without its problems. Indeed, most chemotherapeutic agents are called *cytotoxic*, meaning "poisonous to cells." There is, then, the danger that chemotherapy will damage or even kill healthy as well as cancerous cells.

Because the metabolism of cancer cells is generally higher than that of healthy cells, chemical reactions usually take place much more rapidly in these cells. As a result, the cancer cells take in more of the poison than do healthy cells. Remember, however, that a major difference between cancer cells and healthy cells is their rate of cell division. Cancer cells proliferate more rapidly than healthy cells, but cells in the digestive tract, blood cells in bone marrow, and the cells in hair follicles also grow rapidly. Chemotherapy often damages these normal cells, causing side effects such as nausea, vomiting, and hair loss.

Some side effects of chemotherapy are actually quite serious. Chemotherapy can damage the heart and lungs, lead to infections and ulcers in the mouth, and cause reproductive disorders. According to Dr. Alvin Silverstein, "Even with careful adjustment of the dose, all anticancer drugs have side effects that in some cases may be life-threatening in themselves."

The changing nature of cancer cells limits the effectiveness of many kinds of treatment. Malignant cells can be genetically unstable and when the cancer is advanced, the cells are more likely to mutate, becoming ever more biologically diverse. Furthermore, malignant cells are subject to tumor progression, an increased ability to invade and spread, thereby becoming more difficult to control.

Some cancer cells are inherently resistant to chemotherapy. Some acquire drug resistance as they change over time. Hence the need for multiple drugs used in conjunction or in succession. Efforts to defeat the resistance can, however, cause the resistant cells to proliferate. In addition, a certain kind of cancer cell stops proliferating and escapes destruction through what is known as *kinetic resistance*. In the hopes that one procedure will get what the other misses, physicians and patients often opt for surgery followed by chemotherapy. Some oncologists believe there is no consistent evidence that chemotherapy delays or prevents the recurrence of melanoma after surgery.

Natural Products

Today, several natural products are being used as chemotherapeutic agents. Actinomycin-D, an antibiotic derived from a plant, has been used after surgery and radiation therapy to successfully treat children with Wilms' tumor, a tumor of the kidneys. The cancer seems to occur in the fetus and may not become apparent for years. It is, however, usually diagnosed in children under the age of five.

Other natural products include alkaloids derived from plants. Generally speaking, alkaloids are a diverse and complex group of crystalline chemicals found in plants. Medical researchers have long recognized alkaloids' physiological actions. These chemicals can be analgesic and narcotic; they can stimulate the central nervous system, increase or lower blood pressure, and cause dilation or contraction of the pupils. Among the best known alkaloids are morphine, codeine, ephedrine, and reserpine.

The Greek physician Pedanius Dioscorides used alkaloids from a particular species of crocus in the treatment of cancer.

Scientists today know that the plant Dioscorides used contains colchicine, an alkaloid that is currently used in the production of a treatment for granulocytic leukemia. To this day, alkaloids are providing important anticancer drugs. Vincristine and vinblastine from the periwinkle plant *(Vinca rosea)* are mitotic inhibitors—they prevent cell division (mitosis). These are cell-cycle specific, killing cells by stopping cell division at one particular point. The plant extracts for the treatment of skin cancer that are discussed in Part Three are alkaloids from the plant genus *Solanum*.

The Most Effective Treatment Choices

All of the procedures discussed here are used to one degree or another in the treatment of skin cancer. The most effective treatment depends on which of the three major types of skin cancer an individual has.

According to the American Cancer Society, basal cell carcinoma is a curable form of skin cancer. This is particularly true if the BCC is detected and treated early. Most treatments involve removing the mole-like growths surgically, or removing them with diathermy, curettage, or cryotherapy. In addition, laser surgery and general surgery are often used. Squamous cell carcinomas are routinely treated with surgery.

Malignant melanoma is usually treated with excision. It is essential that lesions suspected of being melanoma not be shaved or treated with curettage or electrocoagulation (hardening of tumors through the application of electrical current). In some cases, lymph node dissection is recommended and partial amputation is sometimes performed. Chemotherapy offers symptomatic relief only. A new immunologic drug now seems a promising therapy for melanoma. Interferon alpha-2B stimulates the body's immune system to defeat the cancer.

Unfortunately, the therapy's side effects—severe flulike symptoms—can be debilitating.

The Danger of Metastasis

Untreated, melanoma cells can spread and form distant tumors in the skin, certain lymph nodes, lungs, liver, brain, and bone. If it spreads, the cancer—which can be detected by physical exam, x-ray, or possibly blood tests—is still considered to be melanoma. Symptoms of metastatic melanoma include weight loss, headache, persistent bone pain, and lumps in the skin.

While melanoma is considered "highly curable" if it is treated early—the survival rate is better than 85 percent—metastatic melanoma is "relatively resistant" to drugs or radiation. Of those whose melanoma has spread far from the primary site, only 2 or 3 percent will survive for five years. If these statistics seem grim, the news gets worse. Most experts believe that a metastatic tumor starts with one single malignant cell that moves from the primary site. Even if 99.9 percent of the malignant cells were destroyed, it might still be possible for a malignancy to proliferate. It is, therefore, essential that *100 percent* of malignant cells be destroyed. Is this possible?

LOOKING TO THE ANSWER

At the moment, risk-free treatment of malignant skin cancers seems like a dream. And with no treatment on which to hang our hopes, we must rely on prevention. Only prevention, it seems, can stem the awful tide of death and disfigurement from skin cancer.

The risk associated with excessive exposure to sunlight is too great to be ignored, and the evidence continues to mount. The intense skin damage caused by sunburns raises your risk of life-threatening melanoma. We must, therefore, stay out of the sun as much as possible. Slapping on a sunscreen and proceeding as if you were impervious to damage is simply not enough. *Remember, sunscreens are not 100 percent effective.* Even on cloudy or hazy days, harmful UV radiation is still reaching you. Umbrellas, which only scatter the sun's rays, do not protect you as well as hats and clothing, which block the rays. Clothing covers you completely and you don't have to worry about reapplying it. And don't think that you can protect yourself by saving your outdoor activities for winter; snow reflects up to 80 percent of the sun's rays.

When all is said and done, your best hope of avoiding skin cancer may be a simple, inexpensive, all-natural preparation. First discovered in Australia and now available in the United States, this preparation may prevent skin cancer—even the potentially deadly melanomas—by effectively treating premalignant skin conditions without significant side effects. The preparation—an all-natural topically applied ointment—has, in fact, been called "the ideal treatment."

In an arena in which current treatments are fraught with negative side effects, high expense, and a high rate of recurrence, this new treatment, which will be presented in Part Three, becomes a very bright beacon of hope.

Part Three

The Answer— Glycoalkaloids

A precious ointment filleth all around about,
and will not easily away; for the odors of
ointments are more durable than those of flowers.

—Francis Bacon

Some of us pluck weeds with a vengeance, regarding them as destroyers of our carefully tended green carpets. But some of us pick dandelions and make wine, while others use cowslip root to make rheumatism tonics. Meanwhile, many animals regard both grass and weeds as a hearty meal. Some animals actually seem to eat certain plants for their therapeutic value. In India and Mexico, for instance, certain varieties of pig eat local plants that are known to fight intestinal worms. Chimpanzees and baboons eat leaves that have medicinal properties, even though they are unpleasant tasting. And in Australia, cows' interest in a certain weed led to a remarkable medical discovery.

In the 1980s, an Australian veterinarian noted an interesting phenomenon among cattle that ate a local weed. When juices from that weed got on the cows' faces, it seemed to halt a cancer that was developing around their eyes. This weed—referred to as Devil's, Kangaroo's, or Sodom's Apple—is *Solanum sodomaeum*. Because the veterinarian had the vision to pick this weed for a purpose, we now have a new spin in the fight against skin cancer.

SKIN CANCER IN AUSTRALIA

It is probably fortuitous that the veterinarian mentioned above lived in Australia—a country so plagued by cases of skin cancer that there is a pressing need to investigate any potential cure or preventative. The skin cancer problem in Australia is, in fact, so severe that two out of three white Australians need treatment for skin cancer by the time they are seventy-five years old. And Queensland, Australia, has the highest rate of melanoma in the world. In 1986, it was estimated that 32 males per 100,000 were victims of the disease. Among white Americans, the rate in that year was 12 per 100,000.

The astonishing melanoma rate in Australia has its roots back in the eighteenth century. The British explorer Captain James Cook reached Botany Bay in 1770 and sailed north to Cape York, claiming that coastline for Britain. Eighteen years later, another Englishman, Captain Arthur Phillip, landed on the coast of Australia and founded New South Wales with just over 1,000 people. Intended as a penal colony, the settlement where Sydney now stands included 717 convicts. Captain Phillip saw great promise in the rich farmland surrounding him on a continent that was largely arid. The captain also recognized the potential for commercial ports in the continent's southeast. Because Captain Phillip encouraged more of his countrymen to emigrate to Australia, the continent was claimed by the British in 1829.

In 1851, gold was discovered in Victoria, bringing scores of

Irish and Scottish settlers "down under." Immigration and prosperity marched forward hand in hand. Eventually, the areas around Captain Phillip's first settlement became the cities of Melbourne, Sydney, and Brisbane—Australia's leading industrial and commercial cities—and Australia became one of the world's great trading nations. But there was a price to pay.

Unfortunately, the original colonists had all been fair-skinned Britons. Their descendants were born south of the equator to parents who had not intermarried with the dark-skinned natives. In addition, during the boom years, darker-skinned Asians had not been permitted to migrate to Australia. This is particularly ironic when one realizes that 20,000 years ago, migrants from southeast Asia settled Australia and became the dark-skinned "natives" or Aborigines.

European colonization of Australia proved costly. Aborigine groups were vastly reduced in number; some became extinct. A recent census revealed that Australia's current population is approximately 13 million, including only 125,000 Aborigines, 45,000 of whom are "pure stock" while another 80,000 have mixed blood. The overwhelming numbers of fair-skinned people who now inhabit the continent have a genetic pool and cultural habits that are not suited to the hot, unrelenting sun. At the equator, about 30 percent of the UV-B rays from the sun reaches the Earth's surface; about 10 percent reaches the tropics and areas further from the equator. Obviously, fair-skinned people aren't suited to life at this latitude. They are paying for their folly in case after case of skin cancer.

Analysis of various data now reveals that the younger a person was upon immigration to Australia, the greater his risk of death from melanoma. This is especially true for those who came from the British Isles, Austria, Germany, and the Netherlands—the most fair-skinned peoples on Earth. Scientists see this data as evidence that exposing fair-skinned children to ultraviolet radiation increases their risk of melanoma.

As a result of its genetic debacle, Australia today has a massive campaign to curtail what had been a growing scourge. "Slip, Slap, and Slop," proclaim billboards as well as magazine and TV ads, imploring Australians to slip on a T-shirt, slap on a hat, and slop on some sunscreen. But what of those for whom the advice comes too late—specifically, those who already have skin cancer or precancerous skin conditions?

Realizing that prevention was not enough, researchers sought answers on every conceivable avenue. When it became known that certain weeds might fight cancer, investigators turned to the plant kingdom for a possible solution.

The search for a completely safe, effective, and inexpensive natural treatment for cancer is not new. Extracts from plants and plant materials have long been used in the treatment of cancers. One of the first people to use plants to treat cancer was the Greek physician Pedanius Dioscorides. The particular species of crocus he used contains the alkaloid colchicine, which is currently being used to treat leukemia. Extracts of saw palmetto are being used successfully in Europe to treat prostate cancer. Once widely used to treat cancer, saffron has been banned for human consumption by the FDA, which says the herb can cause cancer in rats. And at a 1990 symposium conducted by the National Cancer Institute (NCI), soybeans were proclaimed to contain at least five individual anticarcinogens. In addition to being highly efficacious, plant extracts cost about one-third as much as conventional drugs and have few reported adverse side effects.

For more than twenty years, the NCI tested over 100,000 plants as possible cancer-fighting agents. When various extracts were analyzed, some agents were identified that are now well established as antineoplastics (cancer-fighting agents). Among these agents are vinicristine and vinblastine. Both are alkaloids obtained from the Madagascar periwinkle and both are used in the treatment of cancer. Vinicristine has proven especially effective in the treatment of leukemia. In 1983, etoposide—derived from the roots of the May apple—was approved for the treatment of leukemia, lung cancer, testicular cancer, and lymphoma. Then in January 1993, the FDA approved taxol as a treatment for advanced ovarian cancer. This drug was derived from Taxus brevifolia—an evergreen tree known as the Pacific yew (see "Taxol" on page 83).

Another plant often used in folk medicine to treat cancer is *Solanum dulcamara*, which is also traditionally used to treat eye disease, fever, rabies, and warts. The South America Chachi people use it to treat colicky babies. Also known as bittersweet or woody nightshade, this plant was first used by Galen, physician to the Emperor, in A.D. 180. As early as 1825, there were reports in the scientific literature that extracts from *Solanum* plants could be effective in the treatment of cancer.

In 1965, researchers in the Department of Pharmaceutical Chemistry at the University of Wisconsin in Madison experimented with extracts from various parts (roots, rhizomes, stems, leaves, flowers, and fruits) of different plants in the genus *Solanum*. They reported in the journal *Science* that each of the extracts had "significant inhibitory activity" against a certain form of cancer in mice. The researchers subsequently isolated and characterized the alkaloid β-solamarine as an active principle. At that time the researchers said, "The tumor-inhibitory activity of steroid alkaloid glycosides does not appear to have been reported previously." Amazingly, it was rarely reported subsequently.

Interest in *Solanum* extracts resurfaced several years later when their usefulness in the manufacture of drugs was discovered. Diosgenin, an alkaloid obtained from *Dioscorea*, is a precursor in the synthesis of pregnenolone, progesterone, and other medical steroids. Dried rhizomes of the *Dioscorea*, a genus of plants that includes Mexican yams, had once been used for their expectorant and diuretic properties. Because diosgenin was in short supply, alternative raw materials were sought. Solasodine, almost a chemical twin of diosgenin, has now replaced it and may be the sole commercial source of cortisone and progesterone.

Biochemist and medical researcher Bill Elliot Cham, Ph.D., chief professional officer in the Department of Medicine at the University of Queensland in Australia, began experimenting with extracts from the genus *Solanum*, which includes *Solanum tuberosum*, the common potato. Interestingly, this genus of plants gets its name from the Latin word for sun—*sol*. The extracts in Dr. Cham's studies came from the fruit of *Solanum sodomaeum*, the same Devil's apple whose cancer-fighting abilities had been noted by the Australian veterinarian.

The evidence garnered by the observant veterinarian was not the only basis for Dr. Cham's interest. Remember, in 1825, it had been reported in *Elements of Therapeutics and Materia Medica* that *Solanum* extracts were believed to be effective anticancer agents. In 1965, researchers at the University of Wisconsin had reported that *Solanum* extracts inhibited cancer in mice. Yet another research team reported similar findings in 1979. Obviously, Dr. Cham had good reason to be hopeful when he embarked on his project. By 1987, he was reporting in *Cancer Letters*, "Glycoalkaloids from *Solanum sodomaeum* are effective in the treatment of skin cancers in man." Scientists have now identified various plant-based glycoalkaloids, called *solasodine glycosides*, from various *Solanum* plants and have demonstrated their anticancer properties.

GLYCOALKALOIDS OFFER HOPE

The word *glycoalkaloid* is drawn from "glyco" meaning *sugar* and "alkaloid," an organic compound that usually contains one or more nitrogen atoms in a ring. In other words, a glycoalkaloid is an organic compound that contains a sugar and at least one nitrogen atom in a ring containing different kinds of atoms.

Taxol

NCI's researchers began testing samples of yew bark back in 1962. The bark was known to contain alkaloids, chemicals that are often physiologically active. In early tests, extracts of the bark appeared to slow the growth of cancer. By 1967, the researchers had identified the active constituent of the bark—taxol. But because the Pacific yew is very difficult to find, NCI put the project on hold.

In 1977, pressure from the chemists who had worked on the project led NCI to resume its efforts to find out how taxol works. Scientists thought taxol's mechanism of action might be duplicated in the lab. Researchers at Albert Einstein College of Medicine in the Bronx, New York, found that cancer cells treated with taxol stopped dividing. But this promising cancer treatment languished again because taxol is not soluble in water and is, therefore, difficult to administer.

Eventually, investigators tried mixing the taxol with cremophore—alcohol and castor oil—and saline. Patients for whom advanced conventional therapies had failed were treated with the drug. Many became gravely ill and two died from allergic reactions. It seemed that hopes for taxol were doomed until researchers found that the negative reactions were caused by the cremophore, not the taxol. Despite some feeling that the tests were too dangerous to continue, hope prevailed. Test subjects were given steroids or antihistamines to combat allergic reactions, and the taxol was administered slowly over a twenty-four hour period. No more deaths occurred.

Although these trials showed no serious side effects, they showed no significant improvement either. Then, in 1985, an investigator at Johns Hopkins University discovered that taxol did work on ovarian cancer. Testing on women with ovarian cancer revealed that 30 percent of the patients improved; tumor growth was halted and, in some cases, tumors even shrank. Taxol was reported to be six times more effective than the drugs then being used. In January 1991, NCI granted Bristol-Myers Squibb exclusive rights to produce taxol for seven years. In turn, the company would give the drug to the NCI gratis to distribute to physicians while it was experimental.

Finally, in January 1993, the FDA approved taxol for use in women with advanced ovarian cancer. This action opened the door to increased interest in plant-based medicines. Despite this interest, natural therapies are rarely marketed as drugs.

Botanicals cannot be protected by patents or copyrights. Drug companies will not invest millions of dollars in researching a plant and getting it past the FDA unless they can be assured of profit.

Alkaloids are bitter, crystalline substances that contain carbon, hydrogen, nitrogen, and oxygen. Synthesized by the vascular plants and fungi, alkaloids are most commonly found in the leaf, bark, and seeds. Many alkaloids, such as ephedrine, nicotine, atropine, quinine, morphine, caffeine, and pilocarpine, are known for their pharmacological activity. The commonly used anti-cancer drug vinblastine is an alkaloid obtained from Vinca rosa, the periwinkle plant.

Some plants may produce poisonous alkaloids as protection against predators. In other plants, such as rice, the alkaloids function as growth regulators or as reservoirs for nitrogen storage. When alkaloids are consumed by humans, they have a variety of physiological effects. The alkaloid ephedrine, for example, can raise or lower blood pressure. Other alkaloids such as morphine and codeine have been shown to be antispasmodic, analgesic, or narcotic. The alkaloids brucine and strychnine are central nervous system stimulants. One of the most famous alkaloids is quinine, which was the first effective treatment for malaria. Like several alkaloids derived from tropical plants, quinine is antiparasitic.

Because they display such well-established physiological action, alkaloids have been the subject of concentrated scientific investigation. Since 1968, the number of known alkaloids has increased from 800 to more than 6,000. Among these alkaloids is solanine. Because of its narcotic properties, this bitter and poisonous substance was once considered useful in the treatment of epilepsy. Actually a glycoalkaloid, solanine is derived from tomatoes and potato sprouts—members of the genus *Solanum*.

Various plants and fruits from the genus *Solanum* contain glycoalkaloids or steroidal alkaloid glycosides. In addition to potatoes, one of the best known *Solanum* plants is the eggplant. In recent studies, extracts from various *Solanum* plants have been effective against different tumors. In particular, sterol glycosides have been shown to have cancer-fighting properties. Activity against melanoma and ovarian tumor cell lines has been demonstrated with a glycoside known as "solasodine," which can come from any number of *Solanum* plants.

Many glycosides, which are found in abundance in a variety of plants, are therapeutically valuable. These organic compounds yield one sugar and one or more nonsugar substances upon hydrolysis—the reaction that occurs when water is added to a chemical compound. The nonsugar component, called an *aglycone*, is often solasodine, the raw material from which several steroid drugs are synthesized. Steroids, a large family of fat-soluble organic compounds, include certain vitamins, bile acids, adrenal and sex hormones, and natural drugs such as the cardiac stimulant digitalis.

Solasodine must be joined to specific sugars—in other words, it must appear as a glycoalkaloid—in order to fight the growth of a neoplasm or tumor. Preparations that contain solasodine only do not seem to have cancer-fighting ability.

In addition to solasodine, three other glycoalkaloids have been identified as having anticancer properties: β-solamarine from *Solanum dulcamara*, solaplumbin from the *Solanum* plant *Nicotiana plumbaginifolia*, and BEC from various *Solanum* plants—all of which contain solasodine. Solamargine has been shown to be most effective against ovarian cancer, squamous cell carcinoma, choreo carcinoma, Wilm's tumor, and melanoma. The common factor among these anticancer compounds is the sugar component rhamnose, a plant sugar not normally found in mammals. Interestingly, solamargine contains two molecules of rhamnose, whereas some other glycoalkaloids contain only one.

PUTTING GLYCOALKALOIDS TO THE TEST

Faced with a veritable epidemic of skin cancer in Australia, Dr. Cham eagerly set to work formulating a glycoalkaloid-based topical preparation. A cream containing glycoalkaloids was first tested on laboratory animals for five years. In the initial tests, mice with a specific type of sarcoma received single doses of the preparation, which is now called *BEC*. Each dose consisted of 8 milligrams of BEC per kilogram of body weight. Researchers found that the effectiveness of the preparation was dependent on the number of doses, with a daily regimen of three to four doses being optimal.

Survival time of mice given one daily dose of BEC was twenty days. After two doses, 42 percent of the mice were symptom-free. After three and four doses, 92 percent of the test population was symptom-free. Interestingly, when mice were treated with C. parvum, an immuno-therapeutic agent, only 60 percent exhibited inhibition of the same sarcoma. Within weeks, 95 percent of the treated mice were cancer-free and remained so for the duration of their lives.

If the treatment with BEC was effective against the cancer for eight weeks, the mice then lived out their normal three-year life span with no recurrence of cancer. On the other hand, mice inoculated with cells of the same sarcoma but not given BEC generally died within two to three weeks. Although biopsies of the surviving animals did not reveal any cancer, excision of the total area of the tumor site was not always feasible. The possibility of residual tumor could not, therefore, be completely ruled out.

Testing was also conducted to ascertain what, if any, negative side effects might be precipitated by treatment with BEC. Postmortems in the treated mice revealed no obvious signs that could be attributed to toxicity resulting from the glycosides. It was, however, discovered that cytotoxicity can occur when BEC is given at high doses. A single dose with a concentration of 30 milligrams per kilogram of body weight was found to be lethal in at least 50 percent of the test population. Glycosides are known to be inhibitors of cholinesterase, a human enzyme that inactivates the chemical acetylcholine, which is involved in the transmission of nerve impulses. Glycoalkaloids may be toxic, in which case depressed nervous system activity is followed by heart failure and the shutdown of the respiratory system.

The single-dose concentration of 8 milligrams per kilogram of body weight was found to be effective in 50 percent of test subjects. Considering that a single eggplant contains approximately thirty times the amount of glycoside found in a tube of the cream, the danger of toxicity is minimal.

To test for possible genetic effects, the mice that had been treated with BEC were allowed to breed both with other treated mice, as well as mice that were untreated. Six succeeding generations of mice were followed, but no signs of malformation ever became evident, and all the offspring appeared to live normal healthy lives. Furthermore, the litter sizes of treated animals were similar to those of untreated mice.

After many years of working with BEC, Dr. Cham was convinced that it was an effective agent in the treatment of skin cancer. He believed that it could also be used to treat internal cancers. In fact, certain *in vitro* tests have revealed that the preparation is effective against human melanoma and ovarian tumors. Researchers grew melanoma and ovarian tumor cells in a nutrient medium that was subsequently exposed to BEC. Approximately 10 micrograms per milliliter (mcg/ml) of the glycoalkaloid preparation was found to be 100 percent effective against human melanoma and ovarian tumor cell lines.

HUMAN TRIALS IN AUSTRALIA

In his early human trials, Dr. Cham used a solution that contained a mixture of glycoalkaloids, glycosides, and DMSO (dimethyl sulfoxide). A bitter-tasting white crystalline powder, the preparation was called BEC 01.

When the preparation was used, investigators noted rapid tumor regression. There was some suspicion that the DMSO might have been the active ingredient. DMSO is often used to increase absorption of therapeutic agents from the skin, and some researchers claim that DMSO is an effective analgesic and anti-inflammatory agent. There is also some evidence that it can be effective in the treatment of skin cancer. However, a cream containing 10 percent DMSO but no glycoalkaloids could not be shown to have a therapeutic effect on skin lesions.

According to Dr. Cham's protocol for the clinical trials, an antiseptic is first applied to the lesion. The BEC in a cream formulation is then rubbed onto the lesion, which is covered with a bandage. This process is repeated twice a day.

When the cream is applied, there is reddening of the area and erosion or ulceration of the lesion followed by regrowth of normal cells. A slightly painful stinging sensation normally occurs from fifteen to sixty minutes after application. Therapy continues until there is regrowth of skin at the treatment site. The length of treatment varies with the size of the lesion, as well as with the diligence of the patient. Once the cream no longer stings upon application and the area is smooth, the cancer is gone. According to the test protocol, the absence of cancer is confirmed with biopsies. However, it is recommended that the procedure continue in order to ensure a lasting remission.

In clinical studies of patients with keratoses, basal cell carcinomas (BCC), and squamous cell carcinomas (SCC), creams containing 50 percent BEC were well tolerated. Healthy subjects also used the cream and tolerated it well. The best news is that the cream was 100 percent effective in the treatment of solar keratoses, BCC, and SCC.

These controlled clinical trials showed that a mixture of solasonine, solamargine, and certain glycosides was effective against nonmalignant as well as malignant skin lesions. The only side effect was temporary itching or burning around the lesions being treated.

In one controlled experiment, twenty-eight patients with a total of sixty-two cancerous lesions that had been confirmed through biopsy were studied. Two men without lesions were also included in the study as a control. Concentrations of BEC in a cream ranged up to 50 percent, but investigators observed that even 10 percent BEC in a cream formulation was very effective in the treatment of the various skin conditions in the twenty-eight afflicted subjects. No effect was seen when a placebo was administered.

Patients received printed instructions telling them to apply the cream twice a day and then cover the area with a bandage. A fresh protective bandage was applied after each new application.

Patients continued the application until clinical regression was observed (from one to thirteen weeks). The preparation was applied to normal skin in the same manner for eight weeks. Patient compliance was assessed by weighing both the cream and placebo bottles weekly. Because basal cell carcinoma has a small but very real potential for metastasis, it was considered both dangerous and unethical to use a placebo to control experiments involving BCC patients. In this study, only two patients with BCC lesions received placebos. Patients with BCC and keratoses who received the placebo showed mild redness of the lesions. In some cases of keratoses, there was softening and dissolution of the topmost layer of the epidermis. Microscopic exams showed that both the BCC and keratoses treated with a placebo were still present fourteen weeks after treatment had commenced.

With repeated application of the preparation, all the squamous cell lesions responded with rapid softening and sloughing of their crusts. The tissue surrounding the lesions first became inflamed and ulcerated, then healthy skin began to regrow. Patients were considered "cured" within three to eleven weeks. In one case, an SCC lesion on one patient's back had been present for six months. Before treatment it was 20 millimeters in diameter and protruded approximately 10 millimeters. After three weeks, there was an obvious reduction in the lesion's height. After five weeks, histological examination showed that the SCC had been completely eroded.

Thirteen patients with lesions classified as basal cell carcinoma experienced regression in twenty of twenty-four lesions. One patient had two BCC lesions; at the end of four weeks, one of these had totally regressed; the second, which had been very large, was reduced to a quarter of its original size and was successfully excised. In another patient, the lesion decreased in size but the regression was deemed "too slow." Participating researchers believe that the slippery texture of this particular lesion prevented the cream from adhering. Another patient had a BCC on his foot; because it was difficult to use the cream and wear shoes, he withdrew from the trial. Yet another patient stopped participating before regression had been achieved.

Investigators reported that the experiment gave "compelling evidence of the efficacy of the formulation." Complete regressions were observed in:

- 20 of 24 cases of basal call carcinoma
- 5 of 6 cases of squamous cell carcinoma
- 23 of 23 cases of keratoses
- 9 of 9 cases of keratoacanthomas (page 30)

Blood and urine analyses were performed periodically on the trial subjects, and no damage to the liver, kidney, or hematopoietic system (the primary site of blood cell production) was seen. Again and again, the only observed side effects of the BEC cream were mild itching and burning around the treated lesions in some cases. In all cases, outstanding cosmetic results were achieved. Conventional treatments such as surgery or cryotherapy would have caused loss of large amounts of tissue, resulting in scarring. Histological analyses of tissue biopsied before, during, and after treatment confirmed efficacy. After five years, the patients involved in this trial showed no signs of recurrence of cancer. Some patients who were followed for ten years experienced no recurrence.

MORE CLINICAL TRIALS REVEAL EFFICACY

In another study conducted by Dr. Cham, twenty-eight patients with thirty-nine BCC lesions were treated with BEC. Complete regression was seen in 100 percent of the lesions in three to thirteen weeks.

Yet another study involved forty-two females aged forty-two to seventy-one with a total of seventy-two different lesions, and forty-four males aged thirty-eight to seventy-four with sixty-six lesions. All the lesions were at least 5 millimeters (one-fifth of an inch) in diameter and were located on faces, limbs, and trunks. The cream was applied twice a day for three months. Photographic evidence, blood profiles, and microscopic studies of cells in biopsied tissues were gathered. In cases of squamous cell carcinomas, placebos were not used because of the cancer's high probability of metastasis. In other words, the use of a placebo could have actually endangered a subject's life. Complete regression was seen in all of the keratosis patients and in all of the BCC and SCC lesions. Regression occurred in anywhere from three to thirteen weeks. When a placebo was used on fourteen patients with BCC lesions and keratoses for fourteen weeks, no regression was seen. Most of the patients in this study have now been cancer-free for ten years.

In another experiment, twenty-four patients with a total of fifty-six solar keratoses were treated with glycoalkaloid cream. All of the lesions gradually decreased in size until complete regression had occurred. All of these studies indicate that the cream, as Dr. Cham puts it, is "virtually 100 percent effective clinically and histologically" in treating skin cancers.

Summarizing the Trials

In all of the clinical trials, the diagnoses of skin cancer were confirmed by biopsy, and the biopsies were repeated three months after termination of treatment. Blood counts and urine analyses, repeated once a week during the experiment, were all within normal parameters.

With basal cell carcinoma, the order of response to the glycoalkaloid cream was as follows:

1. Initial swelling of the lesion.
2. Redness of surrounding tissue.
3. Ulceration two days later (caused by superficial loss of tissue).
4. Destruction of cancerous cells in three to thirteen weeks.
5. New growth of normal cells.

Response of squamous cell carcinoma to the glycoalkaloid treatment occurred as follows:

1. Rapid softening of lesions.
2. Sloughing of crusts.
3. Inflammation of surrounding tissue.
4. Ulceration.
5. Decrease in lesion size until completely gone in three to eleven weeks.

While efficacy is of paramount importance, there are other significant issues involved in treating skin cancer, the most important being bodily disfigurement. Let's face it, no one wants to choose between health and disfigurement. Fortunately, treatment of all lesions with topically applied glycoalkaloids involves minimal to no scarring. This is quite superior to results obtained with conventional treatments—radiation, chemotherapy, surgery—and can assuredly be considered an advantage. And the cosmetic advantage is not simply a vanity issue; sometimes it's a matter of ensuring a normal life.

Use of the cream formulation to fight skin cancer saved one patient from ghastly cosmetic problems. By the time this patient had gone to see a physician, a basal cell carcinoma had been present on the patient's nose for at least a year. The treatment options were either complete removal of the nose followed by a prosthesis, or treatment with BEC glycoalkaloids. The patient opted to receive treatment with BEC.

During treatment with glycoalkaloid cream, several lesions on the patient's nose ulcerated, and the area appeared to develop into a single large lesion. Because of the ulceration, the cartilage in the nose became visible. After a few weeks of treatment, the nose began to resume its normal shape. Amazingly, after thirteen weeks, the nose appeared normal; tissue biopsy showed no sign of BCC. Furthermore, three years later, there was no recurrence of cancer.

In another case, a BCC on a patient's cheek had been present for four months and was growing rapidly. Treatment with glycoalkaloid cream was accompanied by initial swelling of the lesion and redness in a small area of surrounding tissue. Two days later, the tissue ulcerated. Two weeks after treatment had started, there was a distinct area of ulceration that was actually larger than the original lesion had been. Eventually, there was normal growth of nonmalignant tissue, and after five weeks, a biopsy revealed no BCC.

In 1987, Dr. Cham received permission from Australia's Goods Administration, equivalent to the American Food and Drug Administration, to market an over-the-counter cream for the treatment of keratoses or sunspots. In order to market the cream as a cancer treatment, Dr. Cham would have had to complete additional studies, but he wanted the cream to be available to the public as soon as possible. And the public responded with enthusiasm. In the first year, more than 10,000 units were sold in Australia. The cream, in fact, worked so well, that some in the medical community seemed to feel it was a threat. There was an intense lobbying effort to reclassify the preparation as a prescription item. Now available in Australia by prescription only, the cream was discovered by David G. Williams, D.C., publisher of the widely read health newsletter *Alternatives*. Dr. Williams believes that few prescriptions are being written in Australia because dermatologists and plastic surgeons don't want their patients to know about the cream.

Until Dr. Williams discovered the cream, *Solanum* extracts seemed fated to remain a secret. Fortunately, armed with the information David brought me, I was able to pursue development of an even better, more effective *Solanum* preparation in the United States. This cream is now widely marketed as an inexpensive but effective over-the-counter skin revitalizer.

TESTING GLYCOALKALOIDS IN THE UNITED STATES

Excited at the possibility of a natural, topically applied treatment for skin cancer, I set out to investigate glycoalkaloids derived from *Solanum* plants. Now, I am pleased to report that a team of scientists has developed a new all-natural glycoalkaloid cream. Successfully tested in limited studies in the United States, this cream appears to initiate even more rapid responses than have been seen with the first generation product used in Australia.

A Phase I pilot clinical trial to evaluate the efficacy and safety of the new skin-revitalizing cream was conducted by Margaret Olsen, M.D., a Los-Angeles-based dermatologist. Having spent time in China, Dr. Olsen was "amazed" at how easily Eastern and Western practices were integrated in medicine there. She returned to the United States believing that integration was the wave of the future. When approached about conducting a trial of an all-natural product, she was most receptive.

As fate would have it, an unusual number of patients with actinic keratoses came to Dr. Olsen's office. According to Dr. Olsen, several of these patients were thrilled to be offered something other than chemotherapy. The patients soon began using the all-natural cream that contained *Solanum* glycoalkaloids, as well as sloughing agents and moisturizers. The various ingredients, including extract of willow bark, urea, aloe vera, and menthol, are formulated in a gel base.

Eventually, twenty-three of Dr. Olsen's patients received a four-week course of treatment. All the subjects were fair-skinned blondes or redheads who were extremely sensitive to sunlight. These people had a total of forty-five lesions or regions of actinic keratosis (AK), basal cell carcinoma (BCC), and squamous cell carcinoma (SCC), all of which had been confirmed by biopsy. During the course of the study, the patients rubbed a thick layer of the study cream directly onto the lesion or AK region twice daily. Prior to applying the cream, the subjects were warned to keep the cream away from their eyes. They first removed dead skin or scabbing with a washcloth and cleaned the area with hydrogen peroxide. Once the cream was applied, the area was covered with a bandage. In some patients with AK, the area of involvement was too large to permit total coverage. In addition, many patients found that covering the area was irritating and stopped using a bandage altogether.

During treatment, Dr. Olsen's patients noticed redness, a slight burning sensation, and scabbing on the lesions as well as the surrounding skin. Seven patients reported side effects that included skin peeling and temporary pain ranging from moderate to severe. Five patients reported an allergic reaction to either the occlusive tape or the medication itself. Some of these individuals had experienced similar reactions to topical preparations in the past.

Efficacy of the cream was evaluated using the terms complete response, partial response, stable disease, and progressive disease. Following a thirty-day course of treatment, 96 percent of the lesions showed complete or partial response. BCC and SCC lesions were biopsied again to confirm the absence of cancer.

Dr. Olsen saw the patients every one to two weeks, at which time photographs were taken to document the progress of the treatment. Some of these photographs can be seen in Figures 3.1 through 3.3, on Color Plates Three and Four between pages 102 and 103. The left-hand photo in Figure 3.1 shows a squamous cell carcinoma near a patient's elbow. After seven weeks' treatment with the experimental glycoalkaloid cream, the lesion was completely gone with no scarring, as evidenced in the photo on the right.

A lesion biopsied positive for basal cell carcinoma is shown in the left-hand photo in Figure 3.2. After six weeks' use of a glycoalkaloid cream, Dr. Olsen's patient had regrown healthy pink skin as shown in the right-hand photo.

Dr. Olsen also treated a patient for actinic keratoses. A prescription cream was used on one arm and the all-natural glycoalkaloid preparation was used on the other. Figure 3.3 shows painful red patches after two weeks of treatment to the arm being treated with the prescription drug, while the arm being treated with the glycoalkaloid cream shows no negative side effects. At the end of the treatment, there was no difference in the outcomes, but the patient found the natural product much easier to tolerate.

Nine of Dr. Olsen's study patients had a total of eighteen BCCs. Fourteen of these lesions demonstrated a complete response; that's an astounding 78 percent! An additional two lesions demonstrated partial response, one showed no improvement, and one lesion worsened.

Fourteen people with twenty-five regions of AK participated in the study. In 28 percent of the regions, a partial response was noted. In eighteen regions, a complete response was noted; again the success rate was astounding—72 percent. The rate is even more remarkable when one considers that eight of these patients previously had negative experiences with existing topical chemotherapy treatments. Some had found the burning sensation and pain intolerable. Others found the therapy ineffective. In these eight patients, 67 percent experienced complete responses and 33 percent experienced partial responses.

Dr. Olsen noted some surprising occurrences during the study. One of the patients found that her psoriasis disappeared in areas where she was applying the glycoalkaloid-based cream to treat actinic keratoses. And the psoriasis disappeared even faster than when she had used cortisone. Another observation involved the effect of hairy skin on the action of the glycoalkaloid cream. One patient with very fine, thin hair on the head but thick arm hair experienced a complete response to the keratoses on the scalp but only a partial response to the AK lesions on the arms. Dr. Olsen suspects that the cream can better penetrate where hair is fine.

In summing up the study, Dr. Olsen reported that this cosmetic cream also showed a high degree of topical efficacy for AK, BCC, and SCC. That combined rate of efficacy is an extraordinary 96 percent! Dr. Olsen believes that the treatment is especially good for those with small lesions of actinic keratosis; those that are raised and thick do not respond well. (Such lesions do not respond well to 5-FU or to the frequently prescribed glycolic acid preparations, either.) The doctor also believes that the glycoalkaloid cream is ideal for those who are resistant to traditional therapies.

Dr. Olsen noted that the treatment is most effective for BCCs and SCCs that are covered. The only "downside" she noted was that some people who use the cream for more than a month may develop allergies to it. She also noted that many patients who cover the treated lesions with a bandage find it irritating. She strongly urges patch testing patients for allergy before using the cream, particularly if it is to be used on ankles or legs.

Another study using the same glycoalkaloid cream was conducted by the Plastic Surgery Group of Bloomfield, New Jersey. In this study, eleven patients with various skin lesions were treated with the cream. All of the patients experienced redness, swelling, and irritation when the preparation was covered with a bandage. In each case, the irritation completely disappeared when the treatment ended. Each patient was rated as having a complete or partial response, stable disease, or progressive disease.

In this study, one of the patients with a pigmented lesion on the right arm used the cream for nineteen days, at which time investigators deemed the lesion had undergone a partial response. Another patient with a pigmented lesion on the right arm also experienced a partial response after three weeks of treatment. Partial responses of pigmented lesions of the cheek, chin, right flank, and right upper arm were seen in four additional patients. Yet another patient with a lesion on the left cheek experienced a complete response. Complete responses were also seen when the glycoalkaloid cream was used to treat keratoses, solar lentigo, and a case of squamous cell carcinoma on the neck. The squamous cell carcinoma was gone after thirty-two days of treatment. With one case of basal cell carcinoma on the right shoulder, a partial response was noted after twenty-two days of treatment.

SCIENTIFIC THEORY ADDS SUPPORT

The evidence keeps mounting. In trial after trial, basal cell carcinomas, squamous cell carcinomas, and keratoses disappear when treated with glycoalkaloids extracted from plants in the genus *Solanum.*

All around the world, skin cancer patients are rubbing glycoalkaloid cream on their lesions. Are they fools? Have they been duped into believing that a topical preparation derived from eggplant, potatoes, or kangaroo apples can cure serious disease? Far from it. Because conventional chemotherapeutic agents are often ineffective and always have negative side effects, many researchers, including me, have made it their mission to search for new, less toxic, less invasive, and less brutal ways to combat cancer. Many of these new treatments are plant-based.

Phytopharmacological research—research into the pharmaceutical potential of plants—is burgeoning. One recent survey revealed that more than 1,400 genera of herbs have been used in the treatment of various cancers. Perhaps even more important, ongoing research repeatedly reveals a sound chemical basis for the reputation of these plants. This research is considered so important that the National Cancer Institute (NCI) is involved in a program to screen all the flowering plants in the world in the hopes of identifying some with antitumor activity. To date, approximately 4 percent of the plants studied have shown promise in fighting tumors.

A plant-based cure for cancer is obviously neither fantasy nor science fiction. A topical ointment that can cure skin cancer is no more fantastic. Scientists in the nation's—and the world's—most respected research establishments are working diligently to usher in the day when such cures are commonplace. In November of 1966, one magazine reported, "Researchers have zeroed in on the gene that seems to play a key role in basal cell carcinoma, a common form of skin cancer, and they may develop a cream that can cure it." Indeed, some researchers believe that discovery of the gene called *Patched*, which is involved in skin cancer, "may lead to treatments such as salves or creams."

It appears that the *Patched* gene produces a protein molecule that stops abnormal cell growth. Some researchers now believe that because skin cancer occurs externally, this missing protein can be applied to the surface of the skin to compensate for the faulty gene. Dr. David Leffell, a dermatologist at the Yale School of Medicine, says, "It is not unreasonable to imagine an ointment that, when applied to the skin, may control the growth of cancer." Dr. Leffell said that medications "could be applied directly to the cancer, while minimizing side effects." And Allen Bale, an associate professor of genetics at Yale, says researchers are trying to develop a cream "that will deliver chemicals and proteins to make mutated cells behave like normal ones."

In 1997, the journal *Cancer Letters* included an article written by researchers at the Sree Chitra Tirunal Institute for Medical Sciences and Technology in India. These scientists had conducted experiments in which *Solanum* extracts were given to mice. Approximately 85.67 percent of the test animals had chemically induced skin carcinogenesis. The researchers concluded that application of the extract "significantly inhibited" those cancers to 44.4 percent.

Today, American physicians offer topical treatments only to those with keratoses or superficial BCCs. BCC patients may be given creams containing fluorouracil (5-FU), which fights cancer because it interferes with the synthesis of DNA. Patients using such creams are warned to avoid prolonged exposure to the sun or ultraviolet light, as severe burning can occur.

The topical medication containing 5-FU has several side effects ranging from discoloration of the skin, swelling, soreness, and itching, to the formation of pus. Applications of the cream that contains 5-FU on large ulcerated lesions can be toxic. 5-FU is a cytotoxic agent; it works by killing cells. If too much is used, too many healthy cells are poisoned. We have seen that glycoalkaloids, on the other hand, do not destroy healthy cells. Areas being treated with cream containing 5-FU can be quite unsightly during treatment and for several weeks thereafter. Complete healing can take as long as two months.

One patient who had been using this treatment participated in Dr. Olsen's trial in which glycoalkaloid cream was used. The patient was totally satisfied with the results. While undergoing Dr. Olsen's treatment, he claimed that if he had applied the cream with 5-FU the way he applied the glycoalkaloid cream, he'd be screaming with pain.

Some patients are also given lactic acid creams. Lactic acid is believed to be one of the most effective naturally occurring substances for increasing skin moisture. Dr. Olsen finds that these creams work well for acne and dry skin, but she is "not impressed" by their performance with keratoses.

Now there is another alternative—glycoalkaloid cream—an easy-to-apply cream that is all natural, inexpensive, and relatively free from side effects. Researchers today have demonstrated the effectiveness of glycoalkaloids. In fact, Dr. David Williams, chiropractor and well-traveled medical journalist, reports that scientists using microscopes have actually been able to observe the destruction of cancers treated with *Solanum* extracts. When the war on cancer has been fought for so long on so many fronts with such little success, how can a simple plant extract be so effective?

HOW GLYCOALKALOIDS WORK

Understanding the action of the glycoalkaloids begins with an understanding of cells. On the cell wall of plants can be found endogenous endocytic lectins (EELs). They are called *endogenous* because they originate within the cell. Comprised of protein and a carbohydrate, these compounds are involved in a process of cellular ingestion called *endocytosis*. During this process, the plasma membrane folds inward to bring substances into the cell. EELs bind to specific carbohydrate groups on the plasma membrane of cells and are, therefore, considered receptors for certain sugars. It appears that during carcinogenesis, a number of EELs are present. In fact, some EELs have been biochemically characterized in tumors, including two colon carcinoma cell lines. Investigators think that malignant cells may have more of the receptor EELs than normal cells. This abundance of receptors helps to explain why glycoalkaloids have effective therapeutic effects.

Because *Solanum* extracts have a sugar or glycoalkaloid component, the cell membrane of cancer cells actually brings the

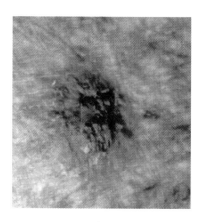 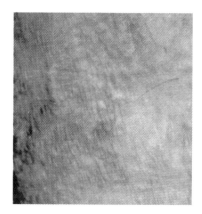

Before   After

Figure 3.1.
The left-hand photo shows a squamous cell carcinoma located near a patient's elbow. The right-hand photo shows the same area after two weeks' treatment with glycoalkaloid cream.

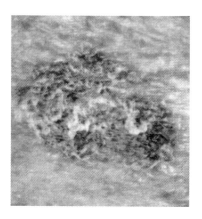 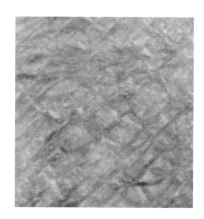

Before   After

Figure 3.2.
The photo on the left shows a basal cell carcinoma located on a patient's arm. After six weeks' treatment with glycoalkaloid cream, the lesion was completely gone, replaced by healthy skin, as seen in the photo on the right.

Color Plate Three

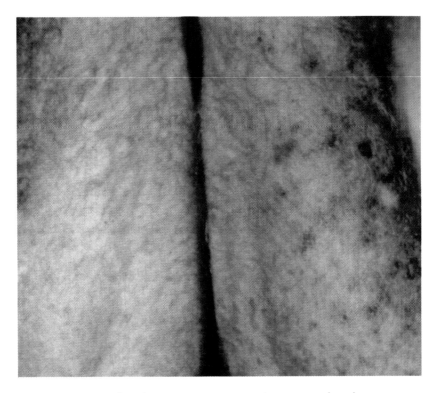

| Arm treated with glycoalkaloid cream. | Arm treated with prescription drug. |

Figure 3.3.

This photo shows the arms of one of Dr. Olsen's patients with actinic keratoses. A prescription drug was used to treat the arm on the right, while natural glycoalkaloid cream was used to treat the arm on the left. The results after two weeks' treatment are shown above.

glycoalkaloid into the cell, thereby opening the door to the destruction of the cancer. When a sugar molecule binds to the EELs or sugar receptors, the process of endocytosis comes into play. The plasma membrane folds inward, bringing the sugar molecule into the cell where it ends up in the lysosome—the part of the cell that contains enzymes used in intracellular digestion.

Using a microscope, researchers have actually been able to see the events that occur after the active sugar component of the glycoalkaloid enters the cell. First, the cytoplasmic membranes rupture. Next, the nucleus contracts and then enlarges. Finally, the nuclear membrane ruptures. When this happens, the sugar compound attacks or ruptures the lysosomes. Because lysosomes are involved in digestion within the cell, when they are injured, the enzymes they contain are released into the cell and literally digest it. The cell simply wastes away.

While individual cancer cells are being eaten away, the active component of the glycoalkaloid is also attacking the mitochondria. Tiny components found in the cytoplasm of cells, the mitochondria are known sites for the generation of energy. They also play an important role in genetic continuity. The glycoalkaloid inhibits the mitochondria's ability to produce energy, thereby disrupting the reproductive cycle of the cancerous cells.

Obviously, there is a clearly defined mechanism of action for the cancer-fighting activity of glycoalkaloids. In fact, in 1990, a report in the well known science journal *Cancer Letters* explained that solasodine glycosides work by bringing about cell destruction or dissolution. The membranes of cancer cells have a receptor for the sugars rhamnose and glucose, which are found in the active component of glycoalkaloids. The compound enters the cell, individual cells are destroyed, new cancerous cells cannot be produced, and the possibility of metastasis or regrowth is eliminated.

It is important to note that neither rhamnose nor glucose alone has any effect on cancer cells. In cell culture, the nonsugar component of the glycoalkaloid did not have a significant effect on ovarian cancer cells. No matter how high a concentration of rhamnose and/or glucose was tested, researchers found no anti-cancer capabilities. However, a relatively low dose of a glycoside derived from *Solanum* killed all of those cells. Remember, glyco-sides yield both a sugar and one or more nonsugar substances. It appears, then, that the *Solanum* extracts are effective in the treat-ment of cancer because of some synergistic or combined effect.

While glucose occurs in most plant and animal tissue and is the major source of energy in the body, rhamnose is rarely found in the cells of mammals. It is, therefore, not likely that normal mam-malian cells would have a receptor for rhamnose. Cancer cells, however, are mutated and might have receptors for these mole-cules. Cancerous cells do, in fact, appear to absorb active glycoal-kaloid components that are not absorbed by healthy skin cells. In experiments conducted in Australia, for example, mice with advanced cancer tolerated very high doses of glycoalkaloids with-out signs of toxicity. In human studies, as well as in cell cultures and *in vivo* animal studies, it was demonstrated that a glycoalka-loid cream has more activity in cancer cells than in normal cells.

Glycoalkaloid cream does not impede regrowth of normal cells when all cancer cells have been killed. It has been suggest-ed that abundant numbers of cancer cells bind with the glycoal-kaloid, reducing its availability to normal cells and rendering it less toxic.

GLYCOALKALOIDS IN THE MARKETPLACE

Glycoalkaloid cream is not considered a drug. As a plant-derived substance, it is classified as a natural product. Sold as a skin revitalizer, glycoalkaloid cream is available in health food stores and pharmacies, and from select dermatologists. When looking for this treatment, be sure glycoalkaloids are listed as ingredients on the label.

Never self-diagnose a suspicious-looking skin lesion. Always seek a qualified health-care provider for a professional evaluation. If you use glycoalkaloid cream, it is recommended that you do so under the watchful eye of your doctor. For additional information on obtaining a glycoalkaloid preparation, see the Resource List on page 123.

LOOKING TO TOMORROW

The cancer-fighting potential of *Solanum* extracts in a cream formula is generating a great deal of excitement. Recent studies have demonstrated that some of these extracts display antitumor activity with human ovarian tumor cell lines, as well as with melanoma cell lines. Ovarian cancer cells were exposed to these extracts, fixed, and examined by Pap smear. Researchers discovered that use of the compounds resulted in approximately 30 percent inhibition. Furthermore, the investigators found they could kill the cancer cells using six to forty times *less* extract than needed with the other cytotoxics investigated (i.e., vinblastine, *cis*-platinum, chlorambucil).

While the hope that *Solanum* extracts can be used to cure a variety of cancers is, as yet, unfulfilled, thousands of patients worldwide attest to the extracts' efficacy in eliminating skin cancers. Their experiences indicate that glycoalkaloids derived from the genus *Solanum* are effective in the treatment of skin cancer at a fraction of the cost of conventional treatments and with far fewer risks and side effects.

Without the groundbreaking work of Dr. Bill Elliot Cham and the vision of Dr. David Williams, the American people might once again have been deprived of a safe, effective, natural treatment. Although information about the effectiveness of *Solanum*

Looking at the Cost of Medicine

Walk into any cocktail party in America and you're bound to hear people discussing the sorry state of health-care and the high cost of medicine. People's dissatisfaction with the pharmaceutical industry is, in fact, helping to fuel interest in alternative medicines.

We are all aware that brand-name drugs are extremely high-priced, and many of us have switched to the less expensive generics. We know, too, that many insurance companies will refuse to pay for brand-name drugs if a generic equivalent is available. But how many of us know why pharmaceuticals are so expensive? How many of us think the price of drugs is simply a case of profit-taking?

One of the reasons drugs, usually fraught with negative side effects, are so expensive is that pharmaceutical companies incur a great expense to evaluate toxicity in order to get drug approval from the FDA. It is estimated that it costs a drug company close to $300 million to get a new drug through the process of FDA approval. Obviously, these companies have to recoup that expense if they are to stay in business.

Although in recent years the FDA has streamlined its drug review times, the Pharmaceutical Research and Manufacturers of America still feel that Americans wait too long for new drugs to become available to them. A study conducted at Tufts University in Boston, Massachusetts, found the decrease in drug approval time has been canceled out by an increase in clinical development time. According to the study, between 1994 and 1995 the average time between the beginning of clinical trials and completion of the application to market a drug was 7.2 years, while in 1990 to 1993 that time was only 5.5 years.

extracts had been published by prominent American investigators more than twenty years ago, no American company had the drive to develop a product. It appears that this is yet another case of reluctance to invest time or money in the development of a natural product.

Although the pharmaceutical industry has long depended on plants as sources of drugs, it seems adamantly opposed to developing and marketing plant products per se. Time and again, pharmacologists and the companies for which they work insist on isolating, identifying, and synthesizing the active ingredient in natural cures so that they can patent their development and reap large profits. Proponents of natural cures must contend with what Dr. Williams calls "modern society's version of the 'Golden Rule,' i.e., those with the most gold make the rules." How sad: The scientists, marketing executives, CEOs, and boards of directors of these companies are just as likely to develop skin cancer as any one of us. Yet they remain too stubborn or too narrow-minded or too greedy to save their own skins. But you can save yours. You can avail yourself of *The Skin Cancer Answer*—the answer that thousands of people already know.

Conclusion

*While allopathic medicine is able to effect remarkable
cures, its focus on cancer, using chemotherapy,
radiation, etc., has been primarily to kill cancer
cells at great expense to the patient's immune system.*

John Prudden, M.D., Med. Sc.D.
Better Nutrition for Today's Living

Skin—we all wear it, but we don't all treat it the same. Some people spend fortunes on their skin, buying every type of cosmetic and antiwrinkle preparation available, while others even have plastic surgery. But many of us virtually ignore our skin.

We spend hours picking out a wardrobe, making sure the clothing fits, the colors match, and the material is appropriate for the weather. We wouldn't dream of wearing anything as wrinkled as we permit our skin to become in ultraviolet light. We would never go out in a storm without an overcoat, but we go out in sun without a protective coat of sunscreen on our bodies.

Clothing is made of fabric: It wears out, we throw it out; it goes out of style, we give it to those whose need is greater. But our skin—the most basic covering we have—is not disposable. It must be cared for and protected, a job Americans—even those who pamper their skin—seem to be doing poorly.

No matter how you treat your skin—whether you devote hours of time and fortunes of money or whether you totally ignore it—your skin is at risk. According to the American Academy of Dermatologists, skin cancer has reached epidemic proportions: More than one million Americans have the disease and the rate is growing by 4 to 5 percent each year. If you have fair skin or red hair, work outdoors, or live close to the equator, your risk is even greater. And sunscreens may not offer the protection we've been led to believe.

Research now indicates that while they protect us against sunburn, sunscreens and sunblocks may not protect us against melanoma, the most deadly form of skin cancer. If it is UV's effect on the immune system that triggers cancer, then protecting our skin against sunburn will not help. So what's a body to do? Better yet, what are you to do for your body?

PROTECT YOURSELF

Be wise about the sun: Avoid prolonged exposure. Cover up with clothing, hats, and sunscreen when necessary. Be aware of blemishes on your body and check them monthly. Be sure to show any suspicious marks to your health-care practitioner, especially if you are in a high-risk group. And if the practitioner tells you that you have keratoses, be aware that use of a topically applied glycoalkaloid derived from the genus *Solanum* can make those marks literally disappear before they can develop into melanoma. Even if your doctor diagnoses the blemishes as basal cell or squamous cell carcinoma, the same glycoalkaloid preparation may protect you from malignancy as well as from more costly treatments and the side effects those treatments entail.

ADVANTAGES OF GLYCOALKALOIDS

Like most of the chemotherapy being administered today, glycoalkaloids from the genus *Solanum* are toxic to cells. However, time and again it has been demonstrated that, unlike other cytotoxic drugs, these extracts have few side effects, none of which is debilitating or even particularly inconvenient. One reason is that an efficacious concentration of the extract is six to forty times less than that of other cytotoxic agents. To understand just how safe *Solanum* extracts are, let's compare them to cisplatin, a widely used chemotherapeutic agent.

It has been demonstrated that *Solanum* extracts' specificity for cancer cells is much higher than that of cisplatin, which means that the extracts attack cancerous cells more than healthy ones. Because cisplatin attacks more normal or healthy cells than do *Solanum* extracts, the drug has far more side effects. Among these are loss of taste, seizures, nausea and vomiting lasting up to twenty-four hours, and renal toxicity. The drug is, in fact, so toxic that the *Drug Handbook* for nurses warns that "preparation of the parental has been associated with carcinogenic, mutagenic, and teratogenic risks for personnel." In other words, those who prepare the drug for injection are subject to the same risks as are the patients. And the risk is not just personal; the drug can cause genetic mutations, which can result in birth defects in offspring.

On the other hand, use of *Solanum* extracts has minimal side effects, consisting of some redness and swelling and occasional pain for fifteen to sixty minutes following application of the cream. The redness is usually followed by erosion, ulceration, dying of treated cells, and regrowth of normal tissue. Although the glycosides in *Solanum* extracts are cholinesterase inhibitors, no complications related to this situation have ever been seen with topically applied *Solanum* extracts. Furthermore, post-mortem exams have revealed no clear-cut symptoms associated with glycoalkaloid toxicity. The glycoside concentrations are simply too low to pose such dangers. The journal *Cancer Letters* reports that the therapeutic index for the *Solanum* extract in the cream being distributed in Australia is "superior to widely used antineoplastics such as vinblastine, cisplatin, and chlorambucil." Patients taking any of these drugs are subject to nausea and vomiting, infertility, and high levels of uric acid in the blood.

The advantages of using glycoalkaloids to treat skin cancer go beyond minimizing side effects. Using the cream is as simple as applying a bandage and changing it once in the course of a day. Treatment with the cream lasts from seven to thirty-five days, depending on the size and type of lesion. Remember, despite the glycoalkoid's ease of use, skin cancer—like any serious disease—should be treated under medical supervision. Only a health-care professional can accurately diagnose the condition and ensure that the disease is truly gone.

In sum, the advantages of using a *Solanum* extract cream over chemotherapy, radiation, or surgery are legion:

- No scarring
- Low cost
- No wound healing
- No surgical risk
- Infrequent recurrence of disease
- Less likelihood that cancer cells will be missed during treatment
- Ease of use

No doubt, there are those who will scoff at the possibility that a completely natural, inexpensive remedy can cure skin cancer. These people are probably totally unaware that many drugs such as aspirin were originally obtained from plants or that the current cancer drug vinblastine is derived from the periwinkle plant. Consider, too, the recent interest in resveratrol, a chemical that occurs in mulberries, peanuts, and grapes, and is believed to have anticancer properties. Reports of this discovery were prominently featured by the media early in 1997 and appeared in the prestigious journal *Science* in January of that year. Few people know that in one experiment, resveratrol was tested on the skin of mice. Mice receiving the treatment developed fewer skin tumors and the total number of mice that developed tumors was reduced. Although natural products are often tested in laboratories, few lay people ever become aware of these experiments. Proponents of what is called "alternative or complementary medicine" have, however, long been interested in natural remedies.

KNOW YOUR OPTIONS

I first stumbled upon the world of alternative medicine back in 1983 when I learned that some of the country's most prominent researchers knew that a substance in shark cartilage could halt the growth of tumors. Much to my dismay, I learned that in more than twenty years, not one of the researchers had ever tried the substance on cancer patients. They were too busy trying to identify the component responsible for shrinking tumors so that they could then purify and synthesize it. This process nets the largest return for pharmaceutical companies. Unfortunately, the dollar sign does figure very prominently in the war against disease today. Consider that an estimated $700 billion is spent each year on drugs, medical equipment, hospitals, doctors, and nurses, as well as such auxiliary services as ambulances. I soon realized that a lot of people stand to lose a lot of money if simple, natural, low-cost therapies and preventatives—the so-called alternative or complementary medicines—became commonplace. And I simply wasn't willing to sit by and permit that situation to remain unchallenged. That's why I wrote my first book, *Sharks Don't Get Cancer,* and why it is currently available in seventeen languages.

Since the book's publication in 1992, I have become an active and vociferous proponent of alternative medicine. You see, I've always been a person who believes the best way to get things done is to take the bull by the horns. You can—and should—live your life the same way. It's important to take your life into your own hands, not be just the flotsam and jetsam tossed about as fate or other people decree.

I remember reading once that Ted Kennedy's son would probably have died of his cancer if he hadn't had such an influential father. Senator Kennedy had all the money and all the contacts to get a warehouse worth of information about the available options. Armed with information about the choices, Kennedy was able to choose the path that saved his son's life. Ted Kennedy took the bull by the horns and prevented his son's becoming a victim of fate, just another statistic.

During my numerous worldwide speaking engagements, I've met thousands of cancer victims who have told me heart-wrenching tales of painful and expensive treatments, crippling frustration, and futility. And I've had to talk to cancer patients and their families knowing full well that the avenues open to them—chemotherapy, radiation, surgery—offer them little more hope than doing nothing at all. With cases of malignant melanoma, "no therapy has been documented that significantly prolongs survival" reported the *California Biotechnology Weekly.* And the American College of Surgeons reports that the overall survival rate for the Stage IV melanoma patients they studied had not significantly improved over the past twenty years.

We would do well to recognize establishment medicine's limitations and become more involved in our own health care. Now that insurance premiums have skyrocketed, now that the costs of medical procedures and prescriptions have become punishing, and now that our government faces the prospect of running out of money to finance this fiasco, we should all start taking responsibility.

We need to learn as much as we can about our health-care options, both alternative and conventional. By reading, by talking with others who have had experience with various therapies, by speaking to health-care practitioners, we can make the informed decisions that will best serve our health-care needs.

Don't let others rule your life. Take responsibility for your own health and well being. Ask questions. Gather information. Make choices. Challenge your doctor to explain "his" or "her" choices. And if you believe that this book has answered more questions than it has raised, you have your skin cancer answer.

Glossary

Alkaloids. Bitter, crystalline substances found in plants; they contain carbon, hydrogen, nitrogen, and oxygen, and most are known for their poisonous or medicinal properties. Their analgesic and narcotic properties can stimulate the central nervous system, increase or lower blood pressure, and cause dilation of the pupils.

Antimetabolites. Substances that compete with or replace a particular product of metabolism.

Antineoplastic. Preventing or inhibiting the spread or development of malignant cells.

Basal cell carcinoma (BCC). The most common form of skin cancer, BCC is a slow-growing malignant tumor that grows up from the basal layer of skin cells.

BEC. A glycoalkaloid cream derived from various plants in the genus *Solanum*.

Carcinogens. Substances having the potential to cause cancer.

Carcinoma. Cancer that develops in epithelial tissue covering body cavities and in the skin or external epithelial tissue.

Chemosurgery. *See* Moh's chemosurgery.

Chlorofluorocarbons (CFCs). Man-made compounds that release chlorine and bromine into the atmosphere; the prime suspect in causing a hole in the ozone layer.

Cryotherapy. Destruction of tissue by freezing it with a probe containing liquid nitrogen. Also called cryosurgery.

Curettage. The scraping off of tissue with a spoon-shaped surgical instrument called a curette.

Cytoplasm. The protoplasm surrounding a cell's nucleus.

Dermis. A second layer of skin cells beneath the epidermis.

Diathermy. The use of high-frequency electromagnetic radiation to destroy cancer tissue.

DNA. Deoxyribonucleic acid; contains the genetic information of a cell.

Dysplastic nevus. A mole that is considered atypical and may degenerate into melanoma.

Epidermis. The outer epithelial layer of the skin.

5-fluorouracil (5 FU). A cancer drug that inhibits DNA synthesis, thereby interfering with cell division.

Glycoalkaloids. Organic compounds that contain a sugar and at least one nitrogen atom in a ring containing different kinds of atoms.

Glycosides. Compounds that can be altered with the addition of water and then yield a sugar and a non-carbohydrate, called an "aglycone." Many glycosides have been found to be therapeutically valuable.

Hydrolysis. Decomposition of a chemical compound as a result of its reaction with water.

Hyperthermia. A method of killing cancer cells by heating blood to between 106°F and 122°F with ultrasound or magnetic induction.

Keratoacanthoma. A rapidly growing but benign raised lesion with hard tissue at its center.

Keratoses. Horny or callouslike growths that appear on the skin. Actinic keratoses, also called solar or senile keratoses, are sharply outlined reddish lesions characterized by thickening and inflammation. They are considered nonmalignant or precancerous. Seborrheic keratoses are benign raised oval lesions that appear yellow or brown.

Laser surgery. Surgical procedures carried out with a tool that transforms light into an extremely intense, small, and tightly focused beam with immense heat.

Lentigo maligna. Precancerous skin lesions that are irregularly shaped, stainlike, and sometimes bumpy.

Leukoplakia. A premalignant condition that occurs on oral or rectal mucosa or on the vulva as raised, whitish lesions.

Lysosomes. Organelles in the cytoplasm of most cells. Bound by a membrane, these organelles contain enzymes that function in digestion within the cell.

Melanin. The substance that imparts color to skin and hair; normally shields skin from ultraviolet radiation.

Melanocytes. Skin cells that produce melanin.

Melanoma. A carcinoma that appears on the skin—usually on the upper back and lower legs—and metastasizes quickly.

Metastasis. The process in which a cancerous cell or cells separate from a tumor and are carried by blood or lymph vessels to a distant site.

Mitochondria. Organelles within cells; they contain genetic material and enzymes important in metabolism.

Moh's chemosurgery. Cancerous tissue is hardened with a chemical and then subsequent layers of tissue are excised until microscopic analysis reveals no cancer cells.

Nanometer. One-billionth of a meter.

Nevus. A congenital lesion or discolored patch of skin caused by pigmentation or by an increase in the number of cells in blood vessels.

Oncogenes. Altered genes that cause normal genes to transform into cancer cells.

Ozone layer. A belt of gasses ten to thirty miles above the Earth's surface that can absorb up to 99 percent of the ultraviolet-B rays coming from the sun.

Patched. A tumor suppressor gene that appears to play a role in basal cell carcinoma.

Placebo. An inactive substance that is used as a control in tests of substances believed to be active.

Protooncogenes. Genes whose abnormal expression can lead to cancer.

Protoplasm. Semifluid, translucent substance that makes up the living matter of plant and animal cells. It is comprised of proteins, fats, and other molecules in a water suspension.

RNA. Ribonucleic acid; responsible for the transmission of genetic information and for synthesis of proteins.

Solasodine. A glycoalkaloid derived from plants.

Solanum. A genus of plants that includes eggplants, potatoes, and bittersweet or woody nightshade. The plants contain glycoalkaloids, some of which have anticancer properties.

SPF (sun protection factor). A measure of protection from sunburn, indicating how long you can stay in the sun without burning. Multiply the SPF by the time it normally takes you to burn. This indicates how long you can stay in the sun without burning.

Squamous cell carcinoma (SCC). A type of skin cancer in which a malignant tumor develops from the layer of skin above the basal layer, the deepest layer of the epithelium.

Steroids. A large family of fat-soluble organic compounds.

Ultraviolet (UV) index. Numbers from 0 to 10 are reported by the National Weather Service to indicate the amount of UV rays that reach a particular area at noon. The higher the number, the more likely you are to burn.

Ultraviolet (UV) light. A type of electromagnetic radiation emitted by the sun. This type of invisible radiation is characterized by the length and frequency of its waves. The range of light that measures from approximately 320 to 380 nanometers (nm) is called UV-A. The range of light that measures between 290 to 320 nm is called UV-B.

Resource List

The following companies and organizations can answer questions and provide information on skin cancer and its treatments:

American Cancer Society (ACS)
"Cancer Answer Line"
1599 Clifton Road, NE
Atlanta, GA 30329–4251
(800) 227–2345
The ACS "Cancer Answer Line" is staffed with professionals who are able to answer questions and provide information on various cancers, patient services, and rehabilitation options.

National Cancer Institute (NCI)
Office of Cancer Communications
31 Center Drive
MSC 2580 Building 31, Room 10A07
Bethesda, MD 20892–2580
(800) 4–CANCER
Provides information on various cancers and their treatment options.

Cartilage Consultants
(800) 742–7534
Offers information on glycoalkaloid cream and other natural cancer treatments.

CompassioNet
PO Box 710
Saddle River, NJ 07458
(800) 510–2010
For information on glycoalkaloid cream and to purchase glycoalkaloid products.

The Skin Cancer Foundation
Box 561
New York, NY 10156
(800) SKIN–490
Provides information on melanomas and other types of skin cancer.

American Academy of Dermatology
930 North Meacham Road
PO Box 4014
Schaumburg, IL 60168
(847) 330–0230
Society of dermatologists that supports research and provides information to the public on various skin conditions.

Bibliography

Adler, T. "Sunscreen Can't Give Blanket Protection." *Science News*, January 22, 1994, pps. 54–55.

Balch, James, MD, and Phyllis A. Balch, CNC. *Prescription for Nutritional Healing.* Garden City Park, NY: Avery Publishing Group, 1990.

"Banned Coolant Is a Hot Item for Smugglers." *Newsday*, January 10, 1997, p. A38.

Burnie, David. *Light.* London: Dorling Kindersley Limited, 1992.

Cham, B.E. "Solasodine Glycosides as Anti-Cancer Agents—Pre-Clinical and Clinical Studies." *Asia Pacific Journal of Pharmacology*, 9, 1994, pps. 113–118.

Cham, Bill E., and Brian Daunter. "Topical Treatment of Pre-Malignant and Malignant Skin Cancers with Curaderm." *Drugs of Today*, Vol. 26, No. 1, 1990, pps. 55–58.

Cham, B.E., B. Daunter, and R.A. Evans. "Topical Treatment of Malignant and Premalignant Skin Lesions by Very Low Concentrations of a Standard Mixture (BEC) of Solasodine Glycosides." *Cancer Letters*, 59, 1991, pps. 183–192.

Cham, Bill E., and Heather M. Meares. "Glycoalkaloids from *Solanum sodomaeum* Are Effective in the Treatment of Skin Cancers in Man." *Cancer Letters* 36, 1987, pps. 111–118.

Cham, Bill E., Merv Gilliver, and Linda Wilson. "Antitumour Effects of Glycoalkaloids Isolated from *Solanum sodomaeum*." *Planta Med*, 53, 1987, pps. 34–36.

Cooke, Robert. "Gene Linked to Skin Cancer." *Newsday*, June 14, 1996, p. A63.

"Curaderm (Antineoplastic) Launched in Australia." *Drug News Perspective*, March 1989, p. 112.

Daunter, B., and B.E. Cham. "Solasodine glycosides. In vitro Preferential Cytotoxicity for Human Cancer Cells." *Cancer Letters*, 55, 1990, pps. 209–220.

Dominguez, Maria, Martina Brunner, Ernst Hafen, and Konrad Basler. "Sending and Receiving the Hedgehog Signal: Control by the *Drosophilia* Gli Protein Cubitus interruptus." *Science*, June 14, 1996, pps. 1621–1625.

Fugh-Berman, Adriane, MD. "Sunscreen or Smoke Screen?" *MS*, July/August, 1994, pps. 19–21.

"The Efficacy and Mode of Action of Solasodine Glycosides (BEC) on Cancer Cells." Proceedings of the Fourth Oceania Symposium on Complementary Medicine, Mark S. Walker, ed., 1993.

Fackelmann, Kathleen. "Melanoma Madness—The scientific flap over sunscreens and skin cancer." *Science News*, Vol 153, June 6, 1998.

"Grape compound with anticancer activity." *Chemical and Engineering News*, January 13, 1997, p. 20.

Hamilton, Virginia. *In the Beginning: Creation Stories from Around the World.* NY: Harcourt Brace Jovanovich, 1988.

Hoffman, David L. "Plants & Cancer Research." Health World On-line, http://www.healthy.net/library/books/Hoffman/Immune /plantsncancer.htm.

Hsu, S.H., T.R. Tsai, C.N. Lin, M.H. Yen, and K.W. Kuo. "Solamargine Purified from *Solanum incanum* Chinese Herb Triggers Gene Expression of Human TNFR Which May Lead to Cell Apoptosis." *Biochemical and Biophysical Research Communications,* 229 (1), 1996, pps. 1–5.

"Iontophoresis of Vinblastine into Normal Skin and for Treatment of Kaposi's Sarcoma in Human Immunodeficiency Virus-Positive Patients." *AMA Specialty Journal Abstracts,* February 24, 1993.

Johnson, Ronald, L., Alana L. Rothman, Jingwu Yie, Lisa V. Goodrich, John W. Bare, Jeannette M. Bonifas, Anthony G. Quinn, Richard M. Myers, David R. Cox, Ervin H. Epstein, Jr., and Matthew P. Scott. "Human Homolog of *Patched*, a Candidate Gene for the Basal Cell Nevus Syndrome," *Science,* June 14, 1996, pps. 1668–1671.

Joyce, Chrostopher. *Earthly Goods: Medicine-Hunting in the Rainforest.* New York: Little, Brown and Company, 1994.

Kenet, Dr. Barney, and Patricia Lawler. *Saving Your Skin: Prevention, Early Detection, and Treatment of Melanoma and Other Skin Cancers.* New York: Four Walls Eight Windows, 1994.

Koutlas, Theodore C., ed. *The Mont Reid Surgical Handbook.* Third Edition, St. Louis, MO: Mosby, 1994.

Kupchan, S. Morris, Stanley Barboutis, John R. Knox, and Cesar A. Lau Cam. "Beta-Solamarine: Tumor Inhibitor Isolated from *Solanum dulcamara*." *Science,* December 31, 1965, pps. 1827–1828.

Kurtzweil, Paula. "Seven Steps to Safer Sunning." *FDA Consumer*, June 1996, pps. 6–11.

Lange, Dianne. "Health: Cancer-Fighting Cream." *Allure*, November 1996, p. 96.

Lapedes, Daniel N., ed. *McGraw Hill Dictionary of the Life Sciences.* NY: McGraw Hill, 1976.

Monhanan, P.V., and K.S. Devi. "Effect of Sobatum on Tumour Development and Chemically Induced Carcinogenesis." *Cancer Letters,* Vol 112, No. 2, 1997, pps. 219–223.

"Monograph on the Compound BEC," *Drugs of the Future,* Vol. 13, No. 8, 1988, pps. 714–716.

Montzka, Stephen A., James H. Butler, Richard C. Meyers, Thayne M. Thompson, Thomas H. Swanson, Andres D. Clarke, Loreen T. Lock, and James W. Elkins. "Decline in the Tropospheric Abundance of Halogen From Hydrocarbons: Implications For Stratospheric Ozone Depletion." *Science*, May 31, 1996, pps. 1318–1322.

MacFarlane, Mark P., James C. Yang, Anshu S. Guleria, Richard L. White, Jr., Claudia A. Seipp, Jan H. Einhorn, Donald E. White, and Steven A. Rosenberg. "The Hematologic Toxicity of Interleukin-2 In Patients With Metastatic Melanoma and Renal Cell Carcinoma." *Cancer,* February 15, 1995, p. 1030.

McAllister, Robert M., MD, and Patricia O'Connell. "The Fine Print." *Skiing,* March–April 1996, p. 32.

Office of Technology Assessment. *Cancer Risk: Assessing and Reducing the Dangers in Our Society.* Boulder, CO: Westview Press, 1982.

"Ozone Hole Diminishing." *Newsday,* May 31, 1996.

Pennisi, Elizabeth. "Gene Linked to Commonest Cancer." *Science,* June 14, 1996, pps. 1583–1584.

Pike, Deborah. "Hot Couture." *Vogue,* April 1994, p. 371.

"Retinoic acid inhibits UV-induced skin damage." *Chemical and Engineering News,* January 29, 1996, p. 24.

Roach, Mary. "The Big Screen." *Vogue,* April 1994, pps. 369–371.

Sabiston, David C. Jr., MD, and H. Kim Lyerly, MD, eds. *Textbook of Surgery: Pocket Companion.* Philadelphia, PA: W. B. Saunders Company, 1992.

Santiago, Lourdes. "PhRMA Chides FDA on Drug Approval Delay." *The Medical Herald,* January 1997, p. 2.

Silverstein, Dr. Alvin, and Virginia Silverstein. *Cancer: Can It Be Stopped?* New York: J. B. Lippincott Junior Books, 1987.

Sinanoglu, Elif. "Wise Up: Don't get burned when buying sunblock." *Money,* July 1994, p. 121.

Sloan, Pat. "UV Index Backs Sunscreen Surge." *Advertising Age,* January 30, 1995, p. 11.

"Study confirms role of CFCs in ozone depletion, researchers say." *Chemical and Engineering News,* February 12, 1996, p. 24.

"Summer Sun Smarts." *McCall's,* June 1995, pps. 34–41.

"Sun? Dial 911." *Mademoiselle,* June 1996, p. 156.

"Sunscreen Labeling to Warn Against Danger from the Sun." *FDA Consumer,* September 1997, pps. 6–7.

"Trial Starts at University of Pittsburgh Cancer Institute." *California Biotechnology Weekly,* June 26, 1995, p. 14.

White, Lisa. "CDC Targets Skin Cancer With Prevention Program." *The Medical Herald,* September 1996, p. 39.

Williams, David G. *The Skin Cancer Cure So Effective, It's Being Kept Secret.* Ingram, TX: Mountain Home Publishing, 1995.

Wu, Corinna. "Melanoma Madness—The scientific flap over sunscreens and skin cancer." *Science News,* Vol 153, June 6, 1998.

Index

plant, 81, 82, 85, 86, 95
Solanum dulcamara, 81
Solanum sodomaeum, 78, 82
Solanum tuberosum, 82
Solaplumbin, 86
Solar keratoses.
Solasodine, 82, 85–86
Solasodine glycosides. *See*
　Glycosides.
SPF. *See* Sun protection
　factor.
Spirocheta pallida, 69
Squamous cell carcinoma
　(SCC), 30, 31–32, 38
　cases of, 22
　treatment choices, 74
　See also Skin cancer.
Steroidal alkaloid glycosides.
　See Glycoalkaloids.
Steroids, 85
Stratosphere, 9
Streptococcus, 65
Strychnine, 85
Sun
　facts about, 4
　minimizing exposure to, 48
　skin aging and exposure to,
　45
Sun protection factor (SPF),
　52–54
Sunburn, 55
Sunscreens, 48–49, 52
　medication and, 52
　skin cancer and, 54–56
　types of, 49, 51–52
　See also Sun protection
　factor.

Surgery
　ancient, 63
　healing after, 67–69
　laser, 60–61
　risks of, 64–66
　skin cancer, 61–63

Tanning
　agents, 44–45
　hazards of, 17–18
Taxol, 83–84
Taxus brevifolia, 81
Textbook of Surgery, 64, 65
Thermosphere, 9
Titanium dioxide, 49, 51
Troposphere, 9

Ultraviolet A (UV-A), 5, 17,
　38, 41–43
Ultraviolet B (UV-B), 5, 9, 17,
　18, 38, 41–43
Ultraviolet C (UV-C), 5
Ultraviolet light. *See*
　Ultraviolet radiation.
Ultraviolet radiation, 5, 41–43
　clothing as protection
　against, 50–51, 57
　minimizing exposure to, 48
　sunscreens and, 49, 51–52
　See also Ultraviolet A;
　Ultraviolet B; Ultraviolet
　C; UV index.
Ultraviolet (UV) rays. *See*
　Ultraviolet radiation.
UV index, 47–48
UV radiation. *See* Ultraviolet
　radiation.

Healthy Habits

are easy to come by—

IF YOU KNOW WHERE TO LOOK!

Get the latest information on:

- better health • diet & weight loss
- the latest nutritional supplements
- herbal healing • homeopathy and more

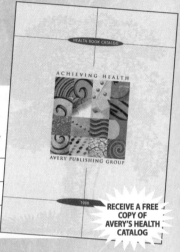

RECEIVE A FREE COPY OF AVERY'S HEALTH CATALOG

COMPLETE AND RETURN THIS CARD RIGHT AWAY!

Where did you purchase this book?

❑ bookstore ❑ health food store ❑ pharmacy
❑ supermarket ❑ other (please specify)_____

Name_____

Street Address_____

City_____State_____Zip_____

GIVE ONE TO A FRIEND ...

Healthy Habits

are easy to come by—

IF YOU KNOW WHERE TO LOOK!

Get the latest information on:

- better health • diet & weight loss
- the latest nutritional supplements
- herbal healing • homeopathy and more

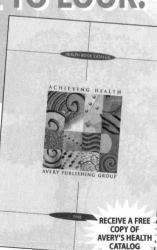

RECEIVE A FREE COPY OF AVERY'S HEALTH CATALOG

COMPLETE AND RETURN THIS CARD RIGHT AWAY!

Where did you purchase this book?

❑ bookstore ❑ health food store ❑ pharmacy
❑ supermarket ❑ other (please specify)_____

Name_____

Street Address_____

City_____State_____Zip_____

Avery Publishing Group

120 Old Broadway
Garden City Park, NY 11040

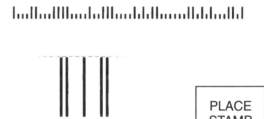

Avery Publishing Group

120 Old Broadway
Garden City Park, NY 11040